For Amy
(

Remember to live life authentically!

Chloe
4.15.07

Getting Ready Chloé-Style

Perfecting Your Authentic Image

Chloé Taylor Brown

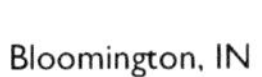
Bloomington, IN

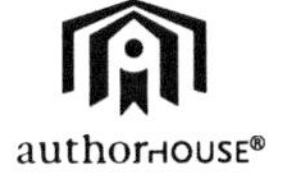

Milton Keynes, UK

AuthorHouse™
1663 Liberty Drive, Suite 200
Bloomington, IN 47403
www.authorhouse.com
Phone: 1-800-839-8640

AuthorHouse™ UK Ltd.
500 Avebury Boulevard
Central Milton Keynes, MK9 2BE
www.authorhouse.co.uk
Phone: 08001974150

First published by AuthorHouse 4/3/2007

ISBN: 978-1-4343-0628-9 (sc)

Printed in the United States of America
Bloomington, Indiana

This book is printed on acid-free paper.

This book is dedicated to Jade, my phenomenal daughter,
whom I greatly admire and love.

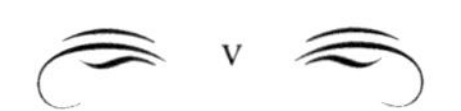

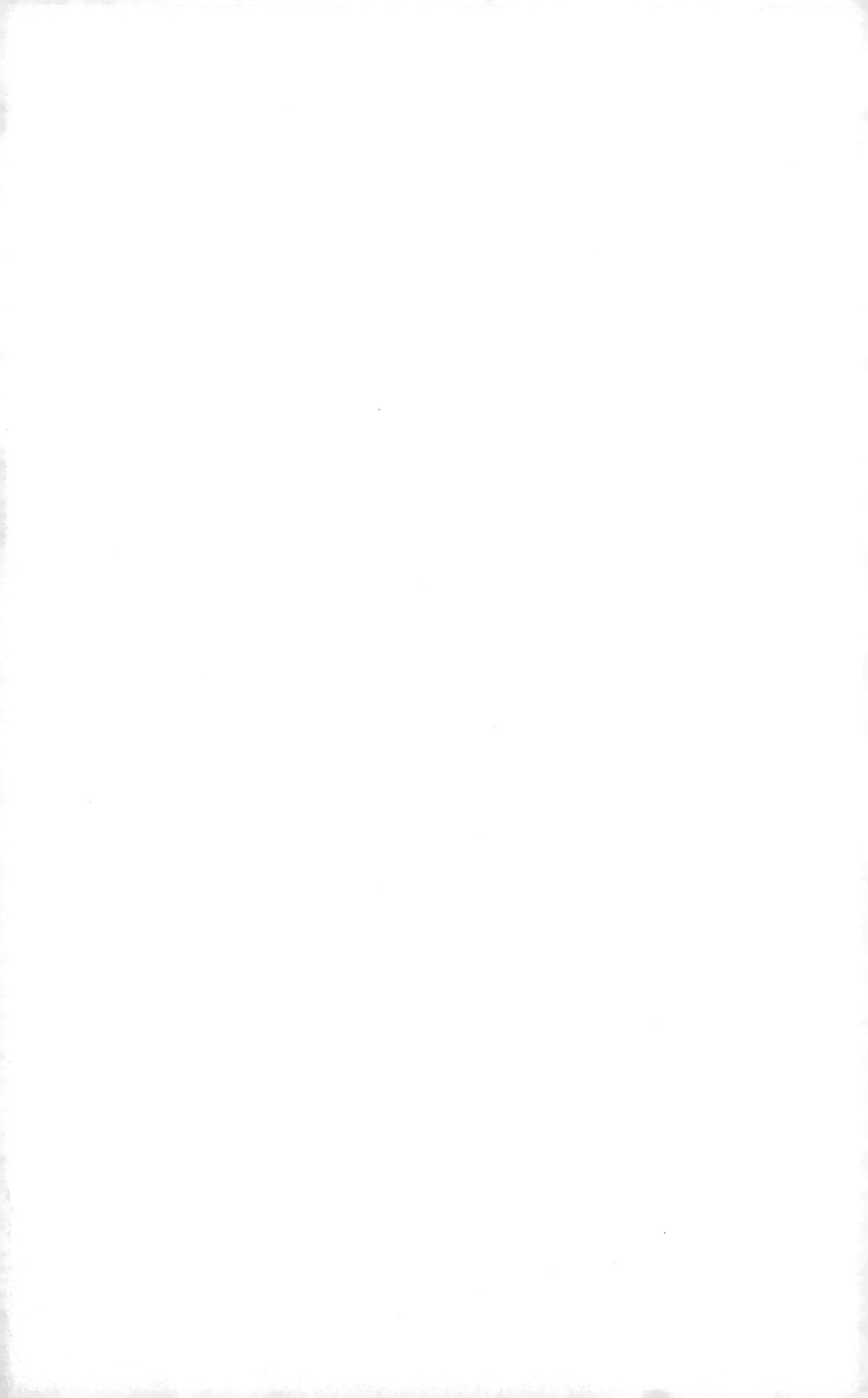

If you want to do something truly wonderful for the world… determine your ideal and make the most of yourself. —Chloé Taylor Brown

Table of Contents

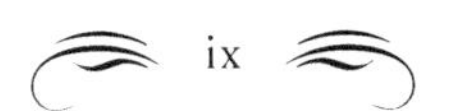

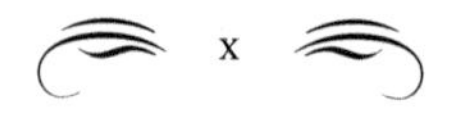

Acknowledgements

This book required the help and support of many individuals, and although I cannot list them all here, I extend my sincerest appreciation to each and every one of them. A few, however, must be mentioned. A heartfelt thank-you goes to Janis Hunt Johnson, my editor, who believed in *Getting Ready Chloé-Style* from the very first pages. I would also like to thank Joan Patrick and Nancy Webster, the two friends who encouraged me to get my message out to the world. To Danny Acres, an amazing photographer, who has the ability through his camera lens to bring out the best in any woman. Thank you to Bruce Jones, my illustrator and fashion designer, for his professionalism, as well as his dedication to fashion and to the creative process. Huge thanks go to my wonderful aunt, Mrs. Anita Walton Moore, for her unwavering support throughout my life, and for her commitment to getting me ready *Anita-Style.* To Auntie Shirley, I'd like to send big kisses on both cheeks, for sharing her beautiful clothes with me after my mother's death. Every writer needs family and friends to encourage her, and I'm blessed with many; I would particularly like to thank my friend and

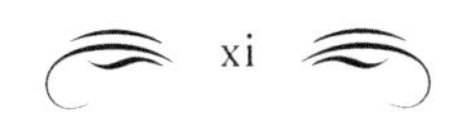

creative mentor Laurie Stieber, for telling me many years ago, "You have a voice, Chloé." Hugs to my sisters—to Angela, for having enormous confidence in me *and* my writing abilities; Brenda, for telling me "I can see it, girl!"; to Cherrie, for talking it up everywhere she goes; and to Normie, my baby sister, for keeping it real. Big thanks to Jade, my amazing daughter, for keeping it fresh and sporty. And finally I would like to thank my husband, Rick Brown, for his love, encouragement and unstinting support for me and for our family. And here's to my boys, Taylor and Joshua, for their confidence that I will one day, cook again. I love you all.

Introduction

You, my darling, are projecting a particular image—everyday, in every way and everywhere you go. It doesn't matter if you are trying to or not. Your image follows you, kind of like your shadow.

Some of us have spent thousands of dollars carefully and meticulously constructing what we believed would be the perfect image for ourselves only to throw it out like yesterday's newspaper and start all over again. Many of us are stuck with images we created for ourselves back in the day, or even images that were created for us by someone else, which may have worked beautifully at the time. Then again, you may be the type who has never put any thought into your image at all; therefore, your image was created for you by default or neglect.

My objective for writing this little book is to inspire and empower you to create an image for yourself and your lifestyle that is completely harmonious with your *true* essence. This is not about a designer suit or the latest pair of fly blue jeans. It is not about the perfect hairstyle—although having a fabulous hairstyle is a good thing. It is not about having more money than you could ever spend, even though that could

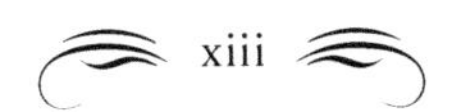

be a good thing for you and for others whom you care about, and even good for the world. But that's not where I'm going with this either.

My purpose for writing *Getting Ready Chloé-Style: Perfecting Your Authentic Image* is to call you to be confident and powerful in all areas of your life and to express yourself authentically—with integrity, substance and style. This can be done by exploring and discovering your true essence, by perfecting your authentic image and by presenting this best image (*your best self*) to the world.

Your visual appearance—the way you present yourself—is important. Please, don't let anyone convince you that the way you behave, look, speak and dress are not germane to who you are predestined to be in the world.

Whatever happened to striving for the more excellent way—the way that helps us to become our personal best?

Your visual presentation can open the most magnificent doors for you. And, darling, the way that you look and act can also get doors slammed shut in your face, never giving you the chance you deserve to express the essence of who you are as a human being and as a woman.

Well, perhaps you have been dying to excavate the most excellent and fabulous you, but you don't know where to start. Or maybe you are so together that you only need a few tips. At any rate, it's perfect timing that you've picked up this book just at this moment.

The title of this book is what I call a real "working title." *Getting Ready* is something that we all do. Most of us do it every day. We get ready for work, for school, the gym, the party, the meeting, and the trial. We get ready for baptisms and for funerals. We get ready for sporting events, as spectators and as participants. We get ready for the beach

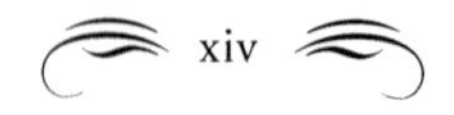

and for weddings; and for hundreds of other occasions. In embracing your individuality, you will begin to realize that you are completely unique. There is no one in this universe exactly like you. You are one of a kind—flawless and beautiful; you *already* have all the qualities or elements that are necessary to be *you*. That's what *perfect* means. Isn't that an amazing realization?

Authentic means being real and true; when you are presenting an image of yourself that is inauthentic or incongruent with who you are, you appear to be fake, untrustworthy and unreliable. For this process to work with integrity you must be genuine, legitimate and completely original. In other words; you've got to be yourself, girl—your *real* self.

Your *image* is simply the way in which you are perceived or regarded. It is a representation of who you are, and many times this representation is not real. It is a public impression. So, then, discovering and perfecting your authentic image is the process of creating and displaying a legitimate, reliable and trustworthy appearance—one that meets the requirements of any occasion.

Who are you really—the authentic you?

Be with that question for a moment because you've got to get this. I want you to determine who you really are. Ask yourself these three questions right now.

1. Who am I?
2. Who do I want to be in the world?
3. What do I want to contribute to the world?

If you don't already know, don't be too quick to answer. Take some time to let these three multi-million-dollar questions resonate. Talk to

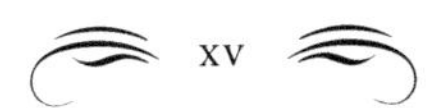

yourself and God about it. Be completely and totally unreasonable. Yes, I said *unreasonable.* So many of us do not become who we are destined to become in the world because we are too busy being '*Ms. Reasonable*' all the time—so think big, bold and beautiful about yourself, darling. If it takes you a while to answer these questions don't worry about it, just don't stop trying until you get *your real* answers. They will be life altering.

Now, I want you to create and perfect an image that is harmonious with the real you. Does that sound difficult? Well, it's not—if you understand the process. How many years of your life have you spent feeling bad about yourself, your intelligence, your skills and abilities, your looks and especially your body? Body image issues are gigantic. Have you ever said, "I am too short, too fat, my butt is too large, my breasts are too small, my nose is too big and my feet are too long; my waist is too thick and my hair is too thin"? This list could go on and on, but now is the time to stop it.

Stop the madness! Step forward, stand tall and break the vicious cycle of negative body talk. This devastates your self-esteem, which for the most part is determined by how you feel about your appearance and how you feel about your body. In order to move forward and reverse the damage society and we ourselves have dumped into our mental and emotional states, we must acquire a new positive way of experiencing ourselves.

Getting Ready Chloé-Style: Perfecting Your Authentic Image is about being your true self, building confidence, setting goals, and understanding the power in projecting your best image at all times. It's about feeling *your* very best—physically, emotionally, spiritually, environmentally and aesthetically, and about living life fabulously.

Once you begin to understand that projecting a poised and polished image while being authentic works for you—your personality, your lifestyle and where you are going in your life—all of the confusion and drama about your appearance will become less complicated. In fact, there will be no *drama* at all. So, come on, get excited about your uniqueness. *I am!*

Part One

You could have everything going for yourself; other people could think you are the smartest, funniest, most beautiful woman in the world; but that's not worth a penny with a hole in it if it's not in alignment with how you think you look and how you feel about what you think.

Chapter 1
Body Image and Self-Esteem

Embrace the uniqueness of your body, your personality and the individuality of your being. The allure and appeal of who you are and how you feel about yourself is embedded within your body image. When you are happy with your body, you feel good about yourself. This thing called body image is an essential aspect of your life and your self-expression. It should never be ignored or made insignificant. Your body image is essentially your power within.

Between the ages of thirteen and sixteen I felt horrible about myself. On a scale of one to ten, I would have rated my confidence and body image about a two or three. First, my mother was tragically killed in an automobile accident, leaving me alone at the very time that I needed her most. Then, it seemed almost overnight I grew to my present height of five feet eleven inches tall. No matter how much Grandmamma tried to fatten me up I could only muster up one hundred and ten pounds—soaking wet. The only body parts that seemed to grow were my hands and feet.

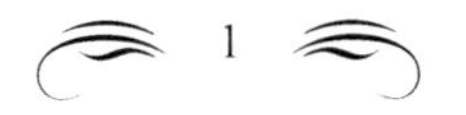

I had horrible posture, none of my clothes fit properly, my hair was a big bushy mess and I wore glasses that always seemed to look crooked. My big feet hung over my shoes while I held on to myself as I walked—as though I would fall over if I let go. Every girl had confidence—except me, it seemed.

Yes, I had big problems, but the picture that I held in my mind's eye of myself was even bigger; it was negative and self-destructive. That's what "body image" is, a picture. That's right; it's like a three-dimensional photograph that we hold in the mind's eye of our body—it's holographic. This perception is psychological, involving our emotions and our imagination. And just when you've become comfortable with hating one thing about your body, something else comes along and you add that to the list. Yes, that picture in your mind's eye is ever changing.

In order to effectively understand body image, it is necessary to first understand that the foundation or the cause of body image lives within aesthetics—in other words, an artistically beautiful or pleasing appearance—and, let's face it, most of us want to be beautiful, or attractive, or at least look good.

You know you like it when someone says to you, "Girl, you look good!"

How you determine beauty and the feelings derived from your perceptions about beauty are subjective. Consequently, body image is a biased view that we make about our own bodies, combined with what we think other people think about our looks and the reaction we get from others. Now, I know all of that sounds crazy, but it's true.

You could have everything going for yourself; other people could think you are the smartest, funniest and most beautiful woman in

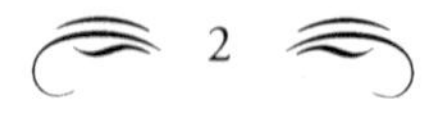

the world; but, that's not worth a penny with a hole in it if it's not in alignment with how you think you look, and how you feel about what you think. It has less to do with your real physical attractiveness and how others see you and almost everything to do with your self-esteem.

***

I am passionate about empowering you to make peace with your body and to begin a proper love affair with yourself. Self-compassion is an absolute must if you are going to move into your true essence, your authentic self. If this is not absorbed and understood, your entire foundation may crack; or it will be shaky, at best. Because your view of your body determines how you treat yourself and how you allow others to treat you—it determines what you can and will accomplish with your god-given gifts. It also determines what you are willing to settle for in life.

Now is the time that we take control of our lives, and it starts with making peace with our innate characteristics, by looking in the mirror and smiling back at ourselves—storing up some self-love. You will be amazed at the warm feelings that bounce off the mirror back toward you. Stop standing in front of the looking-glass complaining about everything that is *wrong* with your body. Build your self-esteem and your self-worth by speaking affectionately toward yourself and about yourself. Compliment yourself on what you believe to be lovely about you and your body. Do this for twenty-one consecutive days and watch your confidence soar.

Being confident has absolutely nothing to do with having a "just right" body. It's about taking care of the body that God has given you and being the best *you* in the whole wide world—especially in your own life, today, right now. Forget about what other women are doing. This is

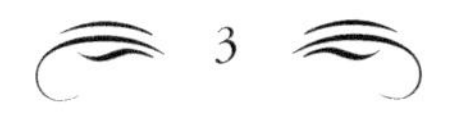

about you, darling, and the good news is it's perfect timing right now. You're not too late or too early to take pride in taking care of yourself. You deserve it—and I know you *can* do it.

Enhancing your body image and feeling good about yourself is essential to becoming who you are supposed to become and discovering and perfecting your authentic image. But, in order to be successful, you're going to need a way to obtain a realistic evaluation of what a healthy body is for you. Allow me to stress how important it is that you understand this concept by asking you to think about the following for a moment. Really! Think about these two questions:

I.What does a healthy body mean to you?

II.What is a healthy body for you?

Before you answer, keep in mind that all of us have a particular body type, shape or silhouette. We have been genetically engineered to have the body that we were born with. Who your parents are and who their parents are have all played a part in what innate characteristics you have acquired. With that bit of information, you can feel free to rid yourself of the notion that there is a perfect body; there is no such thing as a perfect body or a perfect body shape. Each shape has positive and negative traits.

In getting this you will understand why certain fashions and styles look absolutely amazing on you and why you look ridiculous in others. Also, once you see what body type and body shape you have, you will understand what type of wellness and lifestyle maintenance program will work naturally for you.

Chapter 2
Body Types, Shapes and Proportions

Typically, we use the somato type classification system to rate a person's body based on three factors: thinness, muscularity and fatness. The three basic body types are: ectomorph, mesomorph and endomorph—but almost no one is completely one body type or the other. We usually possess elements of all three, with one being more dominant.

In order to feel and look amazing almost all the time it is important to understand your body, its flaws and its assets. And believe me—we all have both, but I'm willing to bet that if you look closely, you'll find more assets than flaws.

I have every confidence that once you understand your body type, your body shape and its proportions you'll be able to see your silhouette in a more favorable light. With a new, positive view of your body, along with your fashion personality type and lifestyle evaluations, you'll learn all the tricks of the trade to look your best authentically—and without putting too much time and energy into the process—because, girl, I know you're busy.

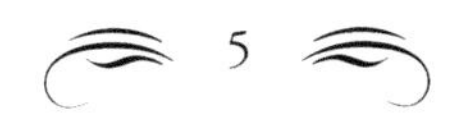

Body Types

The Ectomorphic body type is usually tall and thin with long limbs. I would describe Paris Hilton, Lisa Kudrow and myself as ectomorphs. I am naturally thin; lightly built with a relatively flat chest—with the exception of phases following the birth of my four children. Like most ectomorphs my legs are longer than my torso. I can usually eat as much as I like without gaining weight. If I work very hard and consistently, I am capable of building muscle and strength. However, unlike a true ectomorph, I have good muscle tone and fabulous shoulders. An extreme ectomorph is very fragile and delicate, with light bones, long limbs and drooping shoulders. Many fashion models have this body type.

The Mesomorphic or athletic body type is how I describe Serena Williams, Cindy Crawford and my daughter, Jade, an ACC volleyball player and conference champion. Jade's body is hard and muscular, she has broad shoulders, her chest is medium to large and she, like most mesomorphic body types is extremely strong. Unlike the typical long torso of the true mesomorph, Jade has a short torso. It is relatively easy for the mesomorph to gain muscle mass when training. However, if you have this body type, keep in mind that it may be difficult to lose weight unless you've discovered a fun power sport to take up as a hobby.

The Endomorphic body type is how I describe Raven Symoné, Queen Latifah and Rosie O'Donnell. They are more heavily boned, rounded in appearance, especially around the abdominal area. This body type puts on weight easily in the form of fat and has to work very hard to lose it. Endomorphs' legs are usually shorter than their torsos and they tend to

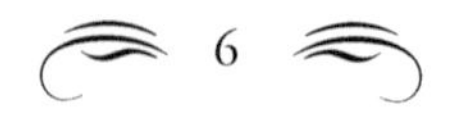

have fuller bosoms than average. If your body type is endomorphic be careful with dieting; the more you diet the more your metabolism slows down—resisting weight loss.

Body Shapes

There are several body shapes, and different charts refer to them by different names, but for the sake of keeping it simple and *Getting Ready Chloé-Style* I am going to discuss six basic shapes: the pear shape, the inverted pear shape, the apple shape, the slender shape, the hourglass shape and the balanced shape.

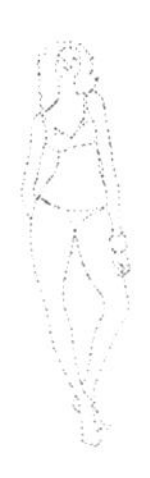

The Pear Shape is the classic female shape. It is characterized by a slim upper body, including slight shoulders and small bust, a small waist and voluptuous hips and thighs. If you gain weight you would more than likely gain below the waist. Your neck may be a beautiful asset.

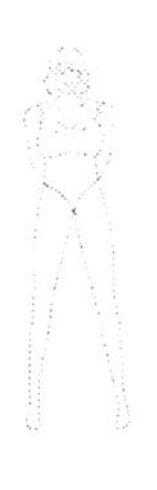

The Inverted Pear Shape is characterized by a larger upper body, with shoulders two or more inches wider than your hips and a large bust accompanied by a narrow lower body. This body type tends to have slim legs and a small bottom with a tendency to put on weight in the mid-section; however, your legs will probably look fabulous forever.

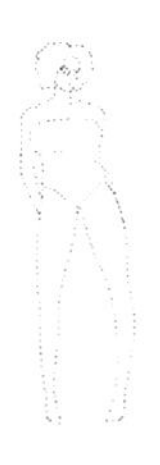

The Apple Shape is characterized as having a top-heavy appearance; your bust and mid-section are bigger and/or wider than your hips. You have a thicker, rounded stomach, abdomen and chest area, with a flat bottom. If you gain weight

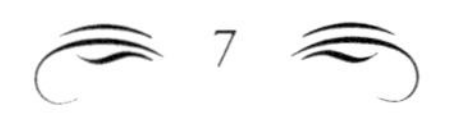

it would probably go right to your top and mid-section. You have nice, relatively thin thighs and legs that will serve you well for a long time.

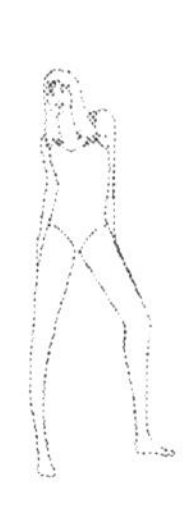

The Slender Shape is characterized as having fairly equal measurements of the chest, waist and hips. You are straight up and down for the most part and may be considered to have an athletic build with slightly broader shoulders. If you gain weight it would probably go right to your mid-section. On the other hand, if you are long and lean then you probably have a high metabolism and will not gain weight easily.

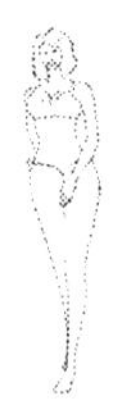

The Hourglass Shape is curvaceous and sought after. The shoulders and hips are balanced with a well-defined waist that could be up to ten inches smaller. If you gain weight though, you will probably gain it all over, from head to toe. Your silhouette is considered to be harmonious and feminine.

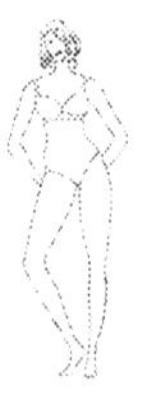

The Balanced Shape is the same size on top and bottom; and, if you are slender your balanced body is the easiest to dress because you can wear almost anything. Most high- fashion designers create designs with your shape in mind.

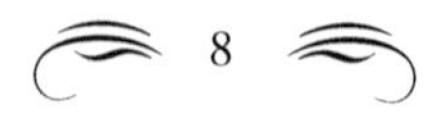

Body Proportions

Consider yourself fortunate if your upper and lower body proportions are somewhat balanced. You have many options in selecting your clothes and putting together a fabulous-looking wardrobe. In fact, the ideal for any body type or shape—no matter how tall or short or how thick or thin—is to look balanced, or to create the illusion of balance.

Height

Your height is certainly a consideration, but it has very little to do with body type or body shape, although we tend to believe it does. On the other hand, when it comes to getting ready and dressing fabulously, you'll want a point of reference.

Petite

You are considered to be petite if you are less than five feet and three inches tall.

Medium

You are considered medium height if you are between five feet and three inches and five feet and seven inches tall.

Tall

You are considered tall if you are between five feet and seven inches and six feet and one inch in height.

Very Tall

You are considered very tall if you are six feet two inches and above in height.

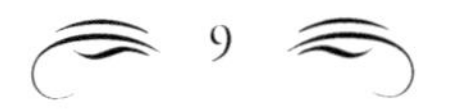

Weight

By now I hope you fully realize that you are uniquely created and that no other *body* is just like yours—you are authentic and there is no reason to compare yourself to anyone. Isn't that good to know?

Yes, we should all know what our *best* body is, how to acquire it and what to do to maintain it. Therefore, the best place to start is by knowing your optimal weight, which is based on your body type, shape, height, body frame size and your age. Know that your body is living and fluid, constantly changing, depending on where you are in your life. Being flexible, patient and persistent are great personal assets in maintaining your weight, which is the foundation for optimal energy and living life fabulously. You'll want to make sure that you are as healthy as you can possibly be. No healthy lifestyle plan is worth its salt if it has given no consideration to a proper diet along with fun, energetic physical activities that get your cardiovascular system racing.

What's your frame size—is it small, medium or large?

You need to know! It will depend on the size and density of your bone structure, your bone mass and muscle mass. Take this simple test to find out what your frame size is.

*Wrap your thumb and middle finger around the smallest part of your wrist.

Ask your doctor to make sure.

•You probably have a small frame if your middle finger and thumb overlap.

•You probably have a medium frame if your finger and thumb touch.

•Your probably have a large frame if your middle finger and thumb do not meet.

The Waist

A woman's waist is not only a consideration in regard to body proportion, it dictates the body silhouette. And more importantly, according to a recent study conducted by *Sister To Sister: Everyone Has A Heart Foundation*, it is to a woman's best health interest to pay close attention to keeping her waist circumference less than thirty five inches. In other words, no matter what body type or shape you have or what size your body frame may be or how tall you are—having a waist line thicker than thirty-five inches means you are in danger of having multiple risks for heart disease and complications from diabetes.

The good news is that with a good healthy lifestyle, including a diet and exercise program, you will have an excellent chance of correcting your waistline. Now, granted, this will not change your body type or your shape, but it will help you to maintain *your best shape.*

Long-Waisted

You are considered long-waisted if your height is in your upper body. In other words—you have a long torso; you are relatively tall but you find that no matter the style of most pants they fit you as though they are a low rise cut. If you are long-waisted you can get away with weighing more without it showing up as unattractive.

Short-Waisted

Consider yourself short-waisted if you have long legs and a short torso; most of the waistbands of your skirts and pants land just under your ribcage.

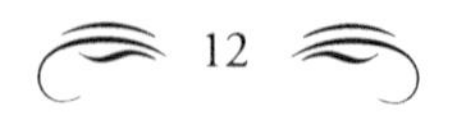

Thick-Waisted

In many cases a thick waist has more to do with your body shape than weight. If your bust, waist, and hips are similar in measurements you would have a thick waist, or if you have an apple body shape then you would probably have a relatively thick waist. At any rate, if you are healthy, you can create curves through the proper selection of body toning undergarments and clothing.

The Chest

Flat-Chested

If you are a woman whose breast did not develop much during puberty and you have very little obvious breast tissue, you are considered flat-chested. But, don't worry, even if you are a 34AA or smaller you can feel and look feminine and fabulous too with the right selection of bras.

Top-Heavy

Consider yourself to be top-heavy if your bra cup size is a DD, a DDD or larger. Problems that arise from being top-heavy can range from poor posture, back pain and finding clothing that looks good with a proper fit. Knowing the proper undergarments to select and where to shop can make all the difference.

Face, Neck and Shoulders

By now you should have a pretty good idea of your body type, shape and figure type, which is critical information when it comes to creating and perfecting your authentic image. Now, it's time to identify your face shape, your neck length and your shoulder shape.

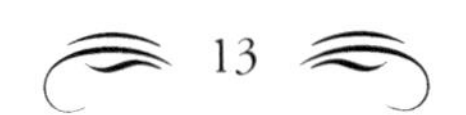

Basic Face Shapes

1. **The Oval** face is slightly narrower at the jawline than at the temples.
2. **The Square** face has a strong, square jawline and equally square hairline.
3. **The Round** face is full with a round chin and a round hairline.
4. **The Heart** face is wide at the temples and hairline with a small chin.
5. **The Triangular** face is an inverted heart shape. It has a dominate jawline and narrow cheek bones.
6. **The Oblong** face is long and slender.
7. **The Diamond** face is a dramatic cross between the heart and oval face shapes. The cheekbones are the widest area, with the jawline and forehead on the narrow side.

Basic Neck Length

1. **A Medium to long** neck
2. **A Short** neck
3. **A Thick** neck
4. **A Too thin and a long** neck

Basic Shoulder Types

1. **Well-defined** shoulders
2. **Full,** rounded shoulders
3. **Uneven** sloping shoulders
4. **Square,** angular shoulders

Chapter 3
The Illusion of Perfection

Earlier I mentioned innate characteristics—unchangeable traits such as your height, body proportions, facial bone structure, the size of your head and feet and a few other traits. It would be a good idea right now for you to begin making peace with these traits. As you start to embrace your body composition, you will learn to accept things about your body type and shape that you cannot change. By making peace with what you believe to be unfavorable characteristics you will become empowered. You will choose to make positive changes in your lifestyle and your self-expression based on self-acceptance.

Because body image is a multi-dimensional concept—we are profoundly shaped by our views and by what we think we see in the mirror—so often what we believe about our bodies just isn't necessarily true. For the most part we hate our bodies in America. In the United States, body dissatisfaction is widespread... and the media, along with the image, fashion and beauty industries have been blamed for their role in shaping perceptions of what is attractive and unattractive about women's bodies.

Yes, that is true—that's what the media does. They take ideas and products that are profitable, or ones that can become profitable, and market and sell them to targeted audiences. That's what fashion advertising has always done, since the inception of *Harper's Bazaar*—America's first fashion magazine in the mid 1860's. In *Bazaar*, the early American designers' gowns were represented by drawings, followed by photography in the 1900's. As the fashion press used more and more photographs of what designers were creating, trends began to spread. At the time, the elite fabulous relied on Parisian designers to maintain their sense of style. The fabulous who could not afford authentic Parisian designs relied on copies from department stores, and for the most part, everyone else designed and sewed their own.

Bazaar, Vogue and *Vanity Fair* were innovators in fashion and advertising. You could say this was the beginning of fashion journalism as we know it today. At the time, these magazines *were* the media; they were promoting American designers and French couture. Designers were the fashion industry, followed by hair coloring companies like L'Oreal and then Elizabeth Arden opening the first modern beauty salon in 1910. Then chic, modern writers made it exciting to read about fashion. Combine this with the social elite of the time and you have the perfect mix for target marketing.

Mass marketing began with the invention of the television in the mid 1950's. When companies realized they could effectively target middle-class suburban families—children, teenagers, housewives and dads—they knew they were on to something big. Fashion advertising has gone right along with all other advertisers; it is an enormous industry. So, most marketers do capitalize on current trends. They say they are only giving us more of what we already want by reflecting the ideals of the current generation.

Get this! The media is massive. The fashion industry is a multi-billion-dollar conglomerate. The beauty business is a one-hundred-and-sixty-billion-dollar-a-year global industry. The diet trade is a multi-billion-dollar industry. Spin-offs from these industries are spas and fitness clubs, diet supplements, diet foods and diet books, not to mention all the diet experts.

These industries are in business to make money, darling, and they are making billions upon billions of it. They are not going anywhere as long as they can keep us hooked into the obsession about our beauty and our weight. That's what advertising is about. It creates a need or desire that you didn't know you had, or it may remind you of something you already knew you wanted or may have had a need for, but you just never got around to buying it. They remind us that we are not good enough the way we are—that we need to do something to make us all right. As a result of them capitalizing on our weaknesses, adolescent girls, college-age women and females in general have become completely confused about what is real in relation to body image, self-esteem and fashion. Because so many of us have bought into the illusion of perfection, we have abandoned our authentic selves. We have been fooled easily, being yanked back and forth and carried about by every new look-good, feel-good potion that claims to recapture youth and make us more attractive and beautiful.

There is absolutely nothing wrong with wanting to look beautiful and feel fabulous. Men and women have sought after beauty since the beginning of time. In Biblical times, the Egyptians saw that Sara, Abraham's wife in Genesis 12:14, was a beautiful and sexy woman.

In medieval times women used bat's blood to acquire a glowing complexion. In the 18th century women used baby's urine to acquire smooth, glowing skin tones. Victorian women were the first to experiment with cosmetic surgery by having ribs removed to acquire a smaller waist to fit in with what they believed to be beautiful.

Looking good matters—it always has and it always will. Attractive people are believed to be more intelligent, to get better jobs, to make more money, to be better lovers, to be more likely to marry and to have more friends. Almost every man that I've interviewed said that having an attractive wife or girlfriend is important; and women also judge other women based on attractiveness. Last, but certainly not least, little babies are more likely to smile longer at an attractive face than at an unattractive one. Beauty has always been a sign of health and fruitfulness. I believe that it is good to seek beauty through wellness, without becoming consumed or driven by it. In order to be authentic, I recommend going deep within to discover your true essence.

Answer these seven life-altering questions.

1. Who am I?
2. Who am I being, right now?
3. What is my personality like?
4. What is my mood level—is it high or low?
5. Where am I headed in my life?
6. Where do I want to go?
7. Am I being *me*, or have I crossed over to being someone else—chasing what someone else has, or chasing every new diet program, beauty cream and fashion trend?

As women, we must do all that we can to understand our own bodies and then choose to create an image based on who we are. When we try to fit into what society wants us to believe is ideal we become confused, striving for an unattainable illusion. Society's ideal is based on distorted

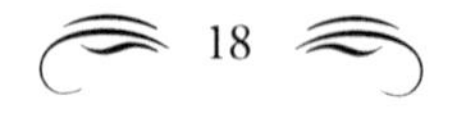

perceptions which, by the way, will change on you just at the moment you believe you have achieved perfection.

Please write down your answers to the seven life-altering questions before moving to the next chapter.

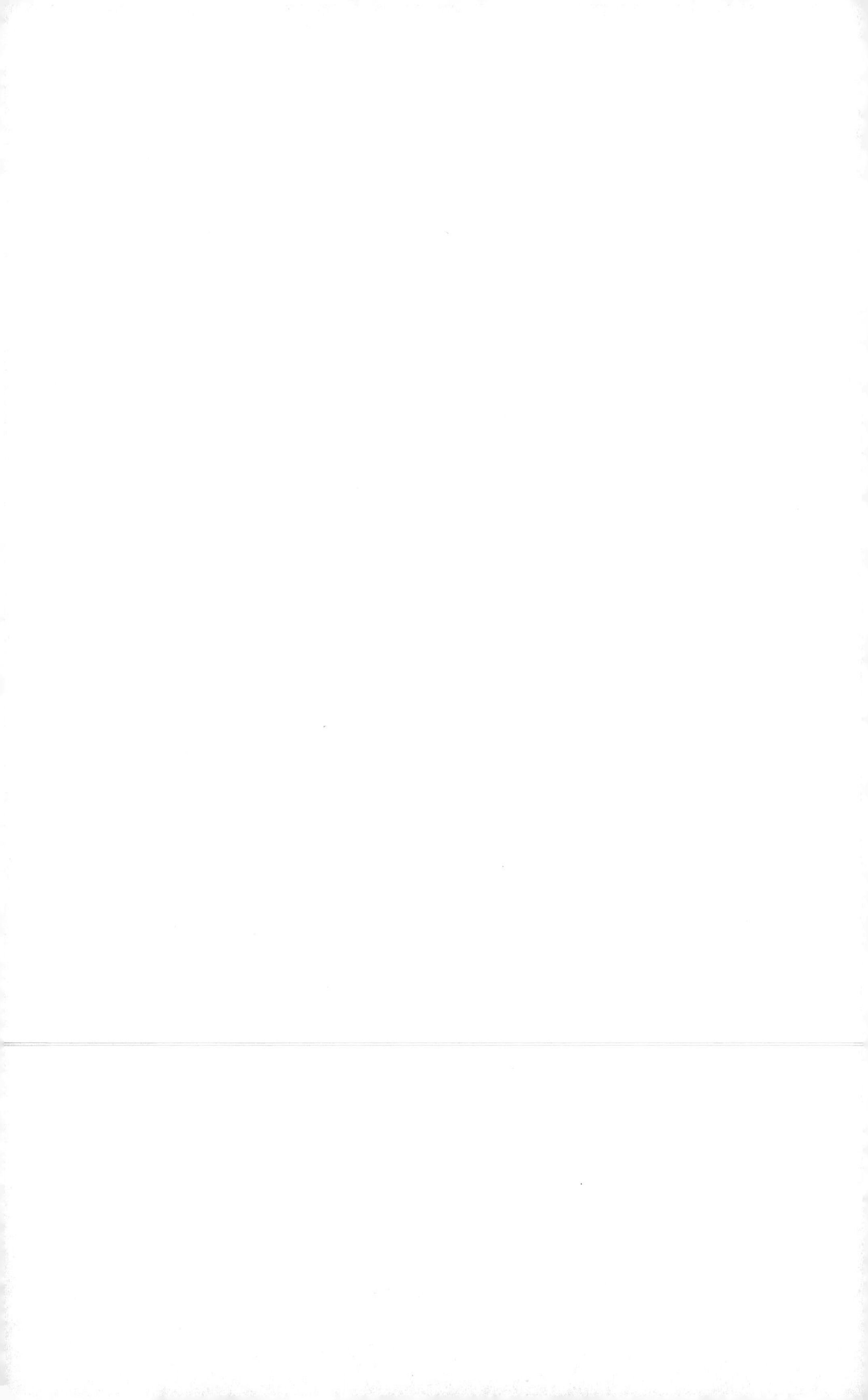

Chapter 4
Changing Ideals—Body & Beauty

Sometimes it is difficult to know where we are going if we do not know where we've been. In regard to the changing ideal body image, we must know that it is cyclical. It may depend on the political state of the country or the world. It may depend on women's movements and other factors. In many cases, it may depend on what men are trying to dictate. As you continue to read this chapter you will see why and how the ideal has changed over the last century.

Everything under the sun has been done.

I think it would be fair to say that the genesis of the media-fashion-beauty connection (MFBC) as we know it today set the standard for the ideal body type and body shape as the mesomorphic-hourglass or curvaceous body. This late-19th-century ideal encouraged women to squeeze themselves half to death by cinching their waist with restrictive corsets; or the worst, removing ribs to fit into the standard of the time. Check out the ideal for subsequent eras.

The 20's Ideal

The mesomorphic-hourglass ideal prevailed until the 1920's, when women were busy inventing new possibilities for themselves and actively pursuing women's rights—political and sexual. These women were gaining social freedom, which was expressed through make-up and fashion. This was also a time when the ideal body type and shape began to shift toward ectomorphic-rectangular or thin and slender.

Women with fuller more voluptuous breasts began to bind them to look flat-chested; obviously, one of the prerequisites for these fashions was a youthful-looking body. Until the 1920's high fashion had been a wealthy woman's pleasure, but the flapper—a shapeless shift dress that emerged from London—changed all of that. The women who wore these fashions appeared audacious; they wore short, sleek hairstyles, boldly applied make-up in public, smoked and danced the night away. Although most women were not flappers, many of us think of this fashion style as being synonymous with the roaring 20's. It was very influential and seemed to fit in with the mood of the early 20's rebellion and freedom.

This was certainly a time of transformation; twenty-six million women gained the right to vote; broadcast radio and the condom were introduced, followed by the first American conference on birth control. Pope Pius XI was outraged by the way women were dressing. But for the first time women were pushing ahead. In 1925 the first women's world's fair was held in Chicago and the first international feminist conference was held in Geneva. Mae West was arrested for obscenity in her Broadway show titled *Sex*.

In 1928 Amelia Earhart made her transatlantic flight. By March of 1929 the New York stock market hit a record high, only to completely crash in October, sending the end of the decade into a very bleak and black mood.

The 30's Ideal

The 1930's eased its way into existence rather depressed. Reckless shopping was over for most; many women made their own clothes or mended and patched the old. The boyish ideal of the twenties was replaced with a return to the more sophisticated ladylike appearance. The mesomorphic-hourglass look was back in vogue. Bust lines were fuller and the waist was very small again. Women had become more productive and busy during the day and as a result they dressed very simply, yet feminine and sweet. The nightlife of these women was all about glamour and sophistication, though. Parisian styles had become too expensive for most of these women. Consequently, American designers began to assert themselves and American fashion started to gain recognition as our foremothers began following the styles of movie stars. This was the time when Hollywood planted its ideals of sex appeal, glamour and beauty into the American psyche.

By the mid 1930's fashion had begun to reflect the mood of the impending war—and by the time World War II actually arrived, clothes were simple, practical and restrained.

The 40's Ideal

During the 1940's, American designers—who had been followers of the French by creating knockoffs—began to take real chances by designing clothing based on the American lifestyle, which was practical, simple and more casual. As a result, their designs and careers began to flourish during and after the war.

America's greatest contribution to fashion—"Ready-to-wear" or *Prêt-à-Porter*, was born during this era. It revolutionized fashion. Now, fashion could be mass-produced and in a finished condition in all styles and sizes, from separates to sportswear and eveningwear. However, because of shortages and rationing of all kinds due to the war, the ideal body shape became leaner again, not as voluptuous as the 30's hourglass. Silhouettes became less adorned, more refined and practical. The fashion look was a boxy square shoulder-padded jacket and short skirts. Some of my favorite fashions were born out of necessity during the Second World War.

A fabulous jumpsuit, originally called the "siren suit" is one of my all-time favorite ensembles—it is whole and complete. With this piece and without much effort you can be as casual or as glamorous as you wish. The siren suit was created to wear over whatever an individual may have been wearing during an air raid in England. Sirens screamed and called citizens to jump into these warm and practical suits and head for shelter.

The wedge sole shoe was created because of a shortage of leather. The cork that was used to construct these shoes turned out to be sturdy and could be worn for miles without making feet hurt, and they lasted a long time, too.

The turban was designed to keep working women's hair in place during the war; but it soon became a way to hide disheveled and uncombed hair. Women were too busy working, running households and doing whatever they could to help out during this difficult time to pay attention to their tresses. Consequently, the turban gave them equal footing—or should I say equal heading.

The 50's Ideal

The 1950's ideal body shape was somewhat thin with a large bust line. A woman's figure and measurements were talked about in magazine stories and in the movies during this time. Today, we talk about pounds and calories; in the fifties, weight was never mentioned—measurements and inches were the expressions.

Indeed, this was an exciting time for fashion and American designers. Women truly wanted to feel and look feminine all over again. They had had enough of the restraints placed on them and their fashions by the war; and because of the ready-to-wear explosion in the forties, fashionable clothes could be found and purchased at all price levels. Like the early 1930's, eveningwear was glamorous, elegant and extravagant. Even though women were clearly preparing to move into a new way of perceiving themselves, they still loved the look of the tightly cinched waist. Daywear was simple yet elegant and the shirtwaist dress was essential to every woman's wardrobe. The average American's standard of living had improved and there was money for all sorts of consumer goods. Yes, the future was looking brighter.

The 60's Ideal

The 1960's were about freedom, creativity, fun and young people and, as a result, the body ideal was girlish and youthful. Baby boomers were coming of age and a woman's image was extremely important. For the first time fashion came directly from the streets. London became the hub of fashion, music and style. Its teenagers had become the emerging fashion voice of the time, and everyone else followed.

Young middle-class kids became the new social elite. They began to rise up and gain social position through fashion design, music, television and film, hair design and make-up artistry. Writers, models and decorators were also included in the young who ruled.

Middle-class suburban families with children and teenagers were beginning to enjoy the finer things in life. And with the introduction of the television—mixed with a strong economy, mass marketing was born. Mass-marketing campaigns were directly targeted toward children and teenagers.

The super-fabulous, super-famous and super-rich Barbie doll appeared on the scene in 1959, and women's perceptions of dolls and of the female form in general have never been the same. Many mothers were apprehensive about Barbie's long legs and arms, large breasts and small waist at first; and rightfully so. But shortly afterwards they seemed to soften, and even to embrace this doll's body—which was not your average baby doll's body! Ironically, Barbie represents the Western woman's ideal... then and today.

I have run into individuals as well as large groups who are angry at Barbie. They claim her "perfect image" is responsible for the large number of girls and women with body-image and self-esteem-related issues and disorders. It would not be fair to assign Barbie full responsibility for the dysfunction of how we as women view ourselves.

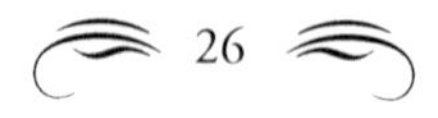

Twiggy, the ultra-slim super model of that era has also been blamed, and as a result there are some who are holding her responsible for our body-image and self-esteem issues and disorders.

Which came first, Twiggy or the mini-skirt?

The mini-skirt became the hottest new must-have for teenagers in the mid-sixties—and just as the 1920's ideal body shape and fashion trend called for a youthful, girlish body, so did the mini-skirt. Women began viewing their bodies disapprovingly, placing a great deal of attention on legs and thighs. The sixties was a turning point in society in many ways, and fashion's impact played a key role.

The media created mass-marketing campaigns that shaped iconic images of celebrities and models in all types of advertisements targeted towards the young. Celebrities began showing up in television commercials and magazine ads sporting the latest asymmetric hairstyles, cosmetics, fashions, and other products that suggested to consumers something was lacking in their lives.

The 70's Ideal

The early 1970's body ideal was a carry-over from the late 60's—young, thin and tomboyish. Many women of the 70's were rebellious and fought against extreme femininity. Consequently, the Women's Liberation Movement embraced this desexualized pubescent ideal and crowned the sexually unattractive Twiggy as the appropriate icon for the movement.

At the time, this ideal seemed good. Women in the Movement were tired of being exploited and wanted the same opportunities as men. Some believed stereotypes of being beautiful and sexually attractive got in the way of their true potential and respect they deserved, so they abandoned make-up and any form of self-improvement or image enhancement, basically letting themselves go. They were proud of the body in its natural state.

The 70's was a time when women encouraged each other to take control of their health and bodies. For the first time since gym classes, women began exercising and paying closer attention to their bodies, especially thighs and buttocks. This fueled the diet, exercise and cosmetic surgery industries. By the late 70's the ideal was thin, and without body fat. A new feminine and still-changing ideal was emerging.

The 80's Ideal

The primary aspiration for so many women during the power-dressing, get-rich-quick eighties was to obtain what they believed to be the "perfect image," which included dressing excessively. It wasn't so easy to acquire this ideal. The 1980's body ideal seemed ambiguous to many. One ideal was the slender but muscular build. Female athletes were making enormous strides while maintaining femininity and athleticism, and they were greatly admired. It was healthy and cool to have a well-toned and well-defined body.

Another body ideal during the eighties was the "super model" image—thin and boyish, or a tubular, slender shape. The eighties super-model was thin, but certainly not a waif-look. The voluptuous hourglass shape was also sought after during this decade, but with less curves on the bottom. Large breasts were in style and many women began

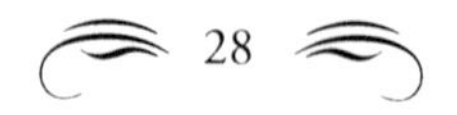

experimenting with breast augmentation and other breast enhancement procedures.

New professional occupations allowed the newly rich to launch lifestyles that one could only dream of in past decades. Women began to make their own money—and lots of it—having a profound impact on the way they felt about themselves and viewed themselves and, as a result, on how they presented themselves to the world. The media and the fashion industry loved it. It appeared that the acquisition of more money brought on bigger shoulder pads, and the bigger the pads the better. There was no such thing as shoulders that were too big. Many women even had their own detachable pads that increased the already professional football-player look.

The pervasive trend that marked this era for each body ideal, though, was "power dressing"—for young professionals and seasoned divas alike. However, by the end of the 1980's the prevailing body ideal became thinner once again.

The 90's Ideal

The early nineties ideal was ectomorphic and slender. This body type and shape projects a pre-teen or waif-look—like that of Kate Moss, who became the 90's Twiggy. The prevailing color or lack of color was black, and grunge spilled into mainstream fashion. The mood suggested a lack of real interest in fashion during the early nineties, which crossed over into corporate America as well. Phrases like "Business Casual" and "Casual Fridays" became part of the corporate vocabulary as many employees began to "dress down."

The prevailing trends were self-expression, individuality and authenticity. Women in Hollywood began to show little interest in "dressing up" and being glamorous; which left the door open for a new breed of fashion divas to emerge. They were Naomi, Linda, Cindy, and several other super models who became household names and kept glamour alive during the early nineties. Society was becoming more urban, and less became more. Silhouettes became neater, jewelry became chic and small, and by the late nineties the ideal body type was even thinner, breasts were big, though, and growing, with the help of breast implants.

Donna, Calvin, Tommy and Ralph ruled fashion during this era. No one could beat the American designers' tactics in marketing and advertising. They knew how to make a woman salivate over what they had to sell. And most of it was in black, except for Tommy's reds, whites and blues. By the end of the nineties the ideal that was projected upon women was clear—extremely skinny, big-breasted and half naked; which led to a multi-billion-dollar diet and exercise industry. Even though American women were spending vast amounts of money to look and feel better about themselves, they became fatter and very dissatisfied with their overall appearance.

The Early 2000's

The ideal body type at the beginning of the millennium was still ectomorphic and slender, or tall and thin with unusually big breasts—a body too thin and too large for most to safely acquire, however. But that didn't stop women from wanting to attain the ideal. This dictated look has continued to fuel women's and girls' insecurities about their bodies, which in turn has continued to stimulate the still-growing diet and exercise industry. Since diets really don't work all that well anyway and many women are not committed to designing and sticking to a healthy lifestyle of eating, moving, breathing and acting properly, out of desperation they resort to nips and tucks to acquire what they have been told is the ideal.

What if we women were to stop chasing this so-called ideal as we know it today and seriously ponder, "Where does the ideal body type or body image come from anyway? Who are the individuals or mega-organizations sitting around making this stuff up?" What happens when we critically assess what resonates within our spirit? I truly believe that because we are already good enough, smart enough and powerful enough, we can change the course of this decade.

Ask yourself, "Why are a handful of powerful industries' prime existences dependent upon me feeling miserable about myself and my body?" If you don't know, consider that it just may be the money in your bank account, or in that designer handbag, darling. They want all of it; and at the end of the day they want you to look in the mirror and still be dissatisfied. If you are, *bingo* for them, because you still don't measure up to this dictated illusion of perfection—and you never will. Americans are fatter than ever and faced with more nutrition, fitness and eating- related health issues than ever before. If we do not rise up and embrace our bodies and recognize who God has created us to *be*, then the future for body-image esteem looks bleak.

Now, because I am an optimist—coupled with the fact that I work to empower females of all ages through natural image enhancement techniques and motivation—I believe that the tides are already turning in how we perceive and love ourselves. The media is slowly beginning to represent women of diversity with different body types, shapes and skin colors in a real and authentic way. But, at the end of the day… it's all up to you and me.

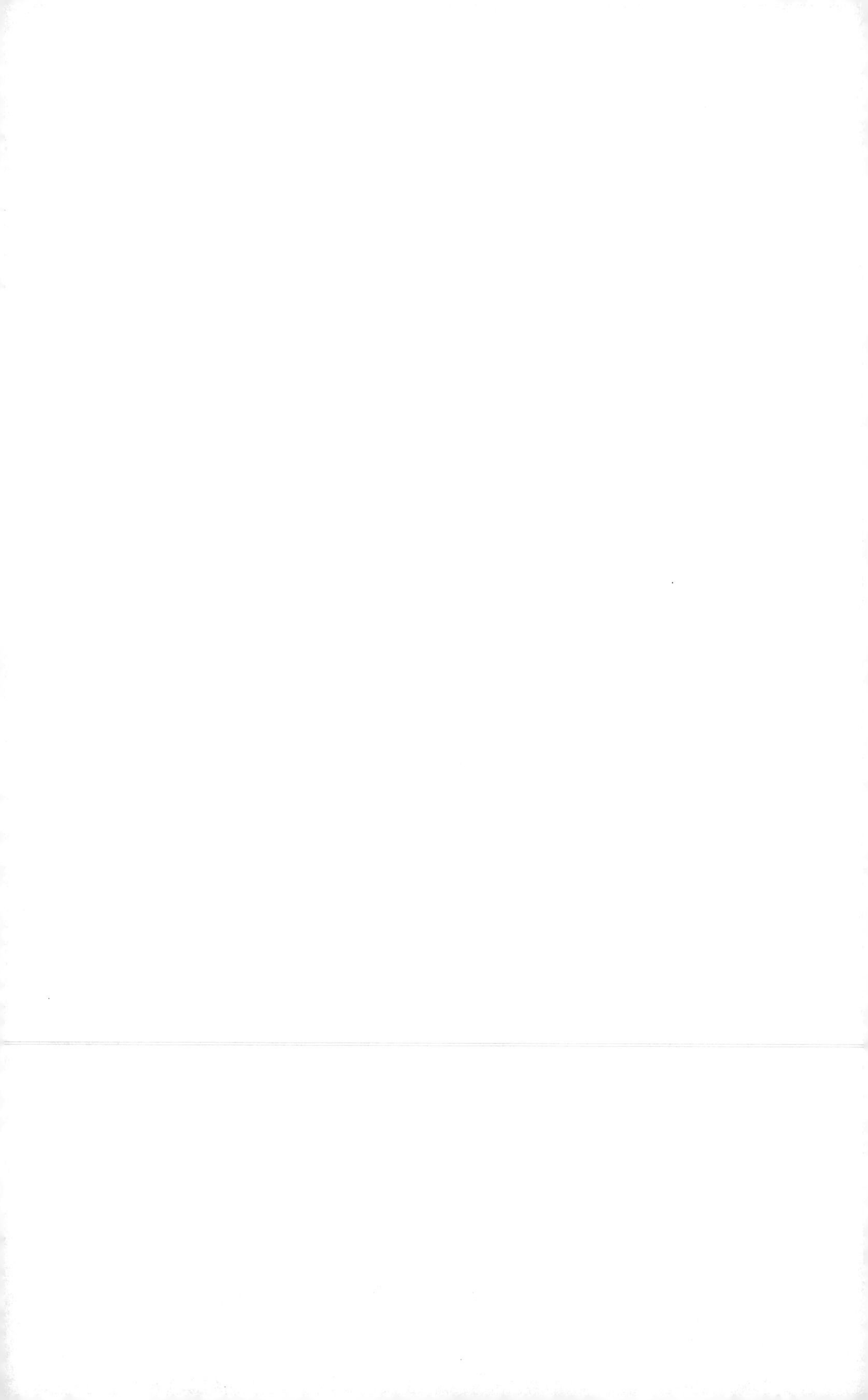

Chapter 5
Creating a Counter-Culture

Based on the history of the MFBC, we will continue to have superficial and unattainable standards of what is desirable and beautiful about women's bodies forced upon us for many decades to come. These messages will no doubt continue to be a thorn in our side.

Unfortunately, many women and girls will give in to the pressure and allure of the slick messages of the MFBC but, the good news is that increasingly, more are rejecting these unrealistic illusions of perfection in search of a more authentic and balanced self. Organizations such as the Eating Disorder Information Network (EDIN) and the National Association to Advance Fat Acceptance (NAAFA) are two organizations doing great work in providing information and support to individuals and groups. I know we can do a better job at bridging the gap between the super fat/obese and the super skinny/anorexic. These individuals are at risk for severe health-related issues, both physically and psychologically. On the other hand, I've worked with hundreds of healthy fat people and hundreds of healthy skinny people. This goes back to body types, body shapes, genetics and hormones and attitude.

The diet industry will relentlessly tell us that we are fat, lazy and self-indulgent.

A clear and concise objective at this juncture for advocates of body-image esteem could focus on education and awareness: Start by providing exciting experiential conferences, workshops, seminars and classes about the "why" behind the MFBC. Demonstrate how to acquire a healthy body and express authenticity. We cannot continue to point the finger at the media or the fashion industry. We must take responsibility by creating an appropriate counter-culture.

When enough extraordinary individuals rise up and stand collectively to expose the media-fashion-beauty connection—the good, the bad and indifferent—then we will begin to make progress. You see, we all, at some point or another have taken the MFBC's messages as a personal attack on us—but it is not personal. As Tiziana Casoli, my Italian modeling agent, told me repeatedly in the beginning of my international modeling career, "it's business, darling."

It is business, darling—a multi-billion-dollar conglomerate of very powerful industries working uncompromisingly and continuously to make money by convincing us that we do not measure up. It's their job. The cosmetic surgery industry will continue to tell us that we are malleable enough to survive any cosmetic procedures and, with a nip or tuck here or there, we can be as beautiful as the most stunning Hollywood celebrities.

The diet industry will relentlessly tell us that we are fat, lazy and self-indulgent and that we will never amount to anything because of our weight—unless we follow their fad diets. Let's face it; we are a nation of overweight people. But, my hope is that we will design a healthy family lifestyle program in which we follow a nutrition and fitness plan for optimal health rather than to lose weight. Looking good and being attractive is important, and there is absolutely nothing in the world wrong with wanting to feel and look your very best—I *am* advocating that. However, designing a plan to be healthy seems to be more attainable and longer lasting than going on a diet to lose weight to look good.

When you experience optimal health your energy increases, your mood level soars, your complexion glows and you feel better about yourself. This makes you more beautiful and confident. Others will notice your confidence, clear complexion, high energy and magnetic mood level and start to compliment you. Their encouragement reinforces the healthy lifestyle that has become part of who you are without much effort at all. This is what I want for you.

The beauty industry will continue to overwhelm us with creams, lotions and corrective serums they claim will transform our lives. Some products claim to de-age, lift and firm—all while you sleep. Others claim to re-surface, repair and recover. *Recover what?*

Please, don't get me wrong, I believe in a proper skin care maintenance régime, cosmetics and other beauty products. They can help us to look better, which usually helps us to feel better. But, at some point we must stop and ask ourselves if we need every new product on the market; and how much de-aging can a topical serum really provide. *Preventive beauty practice* is what I recommend: good nutrition, energetic movement, minimum alcohol, no smoking and living a happy and fulfilled life with lots of laughter.

I have had a great love affair with the fashion industry. For me, it represents my youth, which was filled with excitement, travel, living in Italy, France, Germany and Spain, working international fashion shows where my childhood dream of becoming a fashion model was achieved. To date, it has been the most exhilarating time of my life. Being in the fashion industry, yet having the ability to step back, observe it for what it is and not be *of* it, has been a great challenge. Like any other profession or career, it has high peaks and low valleys.

One of the most important lessons I learned in the business in regard to the fashions and clothes designed is that not every trend and style is for me. And so it is—not every trend and style is for you. Just because the designer introduced it this season does not mean that we have to go out and buy it. When you consider your body type, body shape and lifestyle, you should be able to reject what you know does not work for you. At some point we have to stop blaming the media—although it would be nice if they would take some responsibility. Don't hold your breath. The bottom line is that most of us are very insecure, with low self-esteem and almost no confidence about who we are as women. If we did not have these feelings in the first place, we would not be as easy to influence by a mere picture in a magazine.

Let's develop programs that will foster a strong sense of self in girls and young women.

When we are able to draw from a strong and powerful inner essence, we can love and accept ourselves for who God has created us to be and to become. In being confident, self-accepting, authentic, and poised, we will continue to empower and inform all women and girls about the real meaning of *Getting Ready.*

Part Two

Your appearance is your first communication device and, if used properly, it can be one of your most effective communication tools.

Chapter 6
Image Power & You

The way you present yourself can set you apart and give you power and credibility—or your image can destroy your chances of ever getting through the right doors, not to mention obtaining great success in certain areas of your life. Image is a silent language that speaks volumes. Your image and appearance can be a reliable and legitimate way to present yourself to the world—authentically, or as a persona.

Usually, when we refer to a person's appearance we naturally think of the way she looks or the clothes or fashions she may be wearing at any given time or place. But there is more to it than that. Because fashion, body image and self-esteem are so interconnected, it is essential that you understand that clothing and fashion are often thought of as an extension of who you are as a human being. Now, I know that sounds silly but it is true. Many people look at the clothes and the fashions that you wear as *you* and as a central part of your body image. Because of this, unconsciously, in the body-fashion-self-esteem matrix, you experience something inside of yourself called the *selfing process.*

The selfing process is the communication of the self, which allows you to "*put on.*" This process includes five layers of *getting ready* that work harmoniously together. However, the necessary prerequisites are respecting yourself *and* liking yourself.

The five layers of the selfing process include:

1. Verbal communication
2. Poise, posture and movement
3. Manners and etiquette
4. Grooming and cosmetics
5. Clothing and fashion

In most cases it does not matter which layer of the selfing process you begin to work on first. However, I have found that this process flows smoothly when I follow the five steps as they are listed above.

The selfing process is mainly visual, though it can be tangible, and involve other senses as well.

In understanding how this process works it helps to recognize that bodily behavior and clothing are significant aspects of non-verbal communication, which allows you to create an external identity to present to others.

When you combine the interaction of body image, self-awareness, fashion and communication you can create a mixture of multi-messages.

These messages can easily contradict each other and create confusion for you and for other people watching you. On the other hand, if used

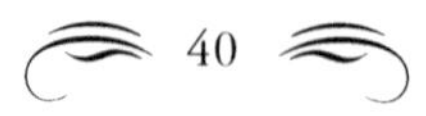

properly, the selfing process can help you to convey messages that are clear and accurate, communication that reflects who you are and what you would like others to perceive about you. You are in control. When creating your external identity it is important to recognize that we are all social persons. No matter how extroverted or introverted we might be, we need to identify ourselves within a group. We all want to *belong* to a certain degree. That's why there are social clubs, organizations, sororities and other groups of interest to individuals. But, in order to belong and be of value, we need to appreciate who we are so that we can share and connect with others. We are also psychological individuals who can be as private and as disconnected as hibernating bears. We are each definitely seeking to establish our individuality as well.

***

Think of a time when you allowed yourself to *put on,* when you practiced the selfing process—a time when you purposely set out to dress and behave in a certain way to accomplish a certain goal. Go on, reflect and write it down.

If you accomplished what you set out to accomplish you projected "Image Power."

In order to acquire and maintain image power at will you must first know, understand and like who you are. Then it's about learning the five steps of the selfing process and putting them into practice. As far as I am concerned, everything about you getting ready and perfecting your authentic image hinges on you liking yourself and the selfing process. Image power has nothing to do with how short or tall you are, how thick or thin or wide or narrow you are. The only thing you need to do is accept *who* you are and create *your ideal image* by following these five steps. You'll know how to be, look and act. You'll be able to go anywhere and fit in and really enjoy yourself. You can look and feel fabulous at any age, height or dress size. Your goal is to accentuate the positives and learn how to enhance your overall image. Don't make creating your authentic image complicated, though. Keep it simple until you feel absolutely sure about your new direction. In the next chapter I'll guide you through each step in the selfing process so you can take yourself there.

Chapter 7
Layers of the Selfing Process

Step One—Verbal Communication

Words are powerful! Knowing the right words to say and when to say them is priceless. But the tone in which you speak and convey your messages, along with your body language, communicate much more about you than words alone. Your tone can convey your mood level and what you are really thinking and feeling. In fact, according to a UCLA study conducted by Albert Mehrabian, verbal communication accounts for only seven percent of how others may perceive you. About thirty-eight percent of how you are perceived depends on the tone of your voice. The largest portion of communication, fifty-five percent, is visual or non-verbal, which falls under the next four steps of the selfing process.

Even though only seven percent of your message is transmitted through words, you had better believe that these words are extremely important. No matter how well groomed you are—if you cannot speak properly, you will not project image power. Instead, you will be perceived as lacking formal education, untrustworthy and even somewhat incompetent.

Recently, as I worked with one of my clients I sensed that something was wrong, even though she had not conveyed this to me verbally. Her body language was incongruent from previous sessions. She assured me that everything was well with her. Not wanting to pry and to maintain professionalism, I took my cue from her and continued with the task at hand as she sat quietly, watching me. After about twenty minutes of us working together she began to tell me what was on her mind, which explained her somber mood.

Based on my client's low mood level, her lack of communication and body language, I knew that all was not well with her, even though, initially, she wanted me to believe otherwise. It was not *what* she said; rather, it was her tone along with her body language that gave her away.

It's important to have the language, words and symbols to express what you feel, believe and want in life. Therefore, don't skip over words that you read or hear in conversations that you're unfamiliar with. Instead, look them up in the dictionary or *Google* them right away—otherwise you'll miss an opportunity to open up a whole new realm of possibilities for yourself through word power. Even if you believe you've been mis-educated you can still learn to express yourself eloquently and effectively with practice. Don't end up being ashamed of looking fabulous… that is, until you open your mouth and out spews mispronounced words used incorrectly—you'll run the risk of losing your credibility.

Ask yourself these questions:

- How is the quality of my voice?
- Can I turn the volume up and down as I please?
- Do I speak too rapidly, leaving others in the conversation to repeatedly ask me to repeat myself?
- Do I speak too slowly, leaving others wanting to complete my sentences for me?

Your Verbal Communication Goals

- To perfect your verbal communication skills
- To come across as intelligent, confident and self-assured
- To be energetic and expressive verbally
- To use colorful words that express your feelings
- To paint pictures with your words
- To make sure your message is not distorted or ignored by using poor diction

Remember to practice by using a tape recorder or video to evaluate your voice.

Step Two—Poise, Posture and Movement

I believe we project our best image when we demonstrate perfect posture, which seems to be a dying attribute these days. When an average woman demonstrates good posture she is revered for her confidence and often her attractiveness. Posture maintenance is a wonderful way to build confidence and feel better about yourself. Your body will love you for it. Your body will begin to show itself off because it feels so much better. Almost immediately you will begin to receive positive responses from others, which will reinforce your behavior.

Posture perfect is more than sitting and standing up straight, although these are important factors to remember. With increased knowledge about your body, good posture can be obtained rather quickly. Good posture relieves tension and strain. It's not being stuffy, stiff or rigid. It helps you to relax into your body's natural positions. Allowing you to move about effortlessly with poise and grace—demonstrating poetry in motion.

Consider these four steps to acquiring perfect posture.

1. **Alignment**—when your body is properly aligned it will move like a well-oiled machine. You will walk and move about painlessly and effortlessly, giving the illusion of gliding. When your body is aligned properly your ears are over your shoulders; your shoulders are over your hips and your hips are over your ankles and your toes point straight ahead. When your body is misaligned you will know it because of tension or even pain.

2. **Balance**—when your body is balanced it equates to wellness. Being balanced means, "knowing one's center" and being able to find it at will. When you acquire a real sense of balance, others will

inquire about your beauty secrets because you will begin to move like a ballet dancer, becoming extremely attractive.

3. **Symmetry**—you must pay close attention to your body and constantly seek symmetry, which is having "balanced body proportions." Your body can become off-balanced or asymmetric from everyday life, like carrying your baby on one hip often. One side of your body may be stronger than the other which affects your balance. If for whatever reason you are asymmetric, fitness training can help by working on distributing strength, flexibility and range of motion equally.

4. **Back Health**—one of the main causes of poor posture is a lack of good back health, and one of the main causes of back pain is poor posture. So, it's time to break the cycle by strengthening and stretching our entire back. Perhaps its time you tried yoga or pilates.

Maintaining good posture is beautiful and functional. It relieves pain, prevents future pain and gives you an air of royal elegance. Try it on for yourself.

Poised, Polished and Perfectly Put Together

When you are poised, polished, and perfectly put together you become more confident about whom you are as a woman and your life goals. Your body image becomes more refined and you acquire that special quality that sets you apart from the average woman. This special quality creates power and credibility for you, providing you with a sense of competence.

In order to maintain poise, you must have the ability to carry your body effortlessly, which means having good posture. Being poised means being self-assured with dignity and composure, like the late Princess Diana, with her elegance and grace: the way she entered and exited from a car—her walk, the clothes that she wore, even her defiance in announcing that she would divorce her husband. She continued to maintain her poise with confidence and grace. But just like the princess, so many of us are not born poised and graceful. Think back to her younger years when she was first pushed into the spotlight by marrying the Prince of Wales. She appeared extremely shy and awkward, not at all like the woman she would become. The point is: There is a princess waiting to be unveiled in each of us.

Movement and Walking Gracefully

Poise and posture can be put to the test by walking. The key to grace and elegance of movement when walking is that it be perfectly natural. Each person has a distinct walk; however, my goal is to help you to relax in your walk, to perfect it through poise, posture and grace. Think of a racehorse. You must learn to move with the same grace, elegance and coordination. Every woman has the ability to walk like a high fashion runway model; it has nothing to do with your height, weight or size, but everything to do with how you feel about yourself and proper training.

As a teenager I felt very uncomfortable and insecure about being five feet eleven inches tall. After years of slumping and stooping, at the age of sixteen Aunt Anita rescued me from bad posture.

"Why are you stooping and slumping?" she asked, truly concerned.

*"I'm too tall," I whined. "Everybody's shorter than me." Aunt Anita knew just what to say, "Only special people get to be as tall as you... your height is bea*utiful."

Her quick and thoughtful response to my insecurities made all the difference in regard to my big body image problems. She was determined to help me feel good about my height and, as a result, I felt better about myself. My height is an innate characteristic that I could do absolutely nothing about. My dear aunt and her friends became my personal image consultants and coaches over an entire summer. When they finished the daunting task of working with me, my whole life changed. My body language reflected a happy and confident young lady as my elegant posture transformed me from what I believed to be an ugly duckling into a beautiful swan. I became poised and graceful, soon receiving many compliments, which increased my self-esteem immensely.

How Are You Being in Your Body?

Complete this little self-examination by performing a standard head-to-toe body check for good posture. The only thing you will need is a full-length mirror—if you do not have one please go out and get one today… every woman needs at least one.

In your birthday suit or undergarments:
•Stand up straight in front of the mirror without bending either knee.
•Make sure you are comfortable with your arms relaxed at your sides.
•Your head should be centered and erect.
•What about your chin, is it parallel to the floor?
•Your shoulders should be at an equal height with your shoulder blades flat and your rib cage high.
•Your stomach should be in.
•Your arms should be slightly bent at the elbow.
•Your buttocks should be tucked in.
•What about your legs—are they straight with both your feet firmly on the ground?

If you are not pleased with the outcome of your assessment—for instance, if you're holding on to yourself or shifting all of your weight to one leg, or your head is tilting to one side, or perhaps your shoulders are curved—then you must modify your position to bring it into line with these posture-perfect suggestions. Have a family member or friend watch and encourage you as you practice and they videotape you. That way you can see for yourself what you may need to work on to improve your posture. Once you are comfortable with your posture, you'll be ready to take the next step. Literally, just take the next step and begin walking. Until you become absolutely sure that you have *the model's walk,* continue to practice to both your favorite upbeat and slow music at least 30 minutes each day. *Don't forget to critique the videotape.*

Gestures Speak Volumes

When your verbal communication is untruthful your non-verbal communication, gestures or body language may give you away as a liar. Gestures can be a wonderful way to assist you in communicating your feelings and what you are thinking. They can help make your conversations more animated and exciting. However, it is also important to realize that gestures can be misleading if you do not have body awareness.

Your gestures and movement should match the situation at hand. If you are having a conversation with a friend, giving her the best news of your life and she responds by screaming and crying with an angry look on her face while telling you how happy she is for you, then something is wrong with that picture. Her words, body language and actions don't add up. Facial expressions can be a dead give-away, conveying exactly what you may be thinking or feeling, which, in many situations, could be offensive to others. Some gestures and facial expressions are culturally specific, but there are some emotions that are expressed the same way, regardless of cultural differences. These universal emotions are happiness, sadness, fear, anger, surprise, embarrassment and disgust. It would be wise to study your facial expressions so as not to offend others, or so that you can maintain the upper hand in certain situations.

The all-time universal facial expression is a smile.

A true smile can reveal happiness and joy. The corners of your mouth will curve upward; your eyes will twinkle causing the outer corners to crinkle into crow's feet. Divas... don't worry. These crow's feet are a good thing. This type of heartfelt smile is difficult to produce on demand. It is controlled by your emotions and it is a true reflection of your mood level. However, with body awareness you can use your facial expressions to maintain the upper hand, dictating how you want others to perceive you.

In only a few situations would a smile be inappropriate. In most situations, a smile can change the mood by putting others at ease and letting them know that you are friendly and enjoying their company. Don't forget to make the appropriate eye contact. Too much eye contact is intimidating and not enough sends the message that you are insecure or have something to hide. In a typical conversation, the speaker makes eye contact about forty percent of the time and the listener generally makes eye contact about seventy percent of the time. Use your good judgment to adjust your eye contact for the situation at hand.

Step Three—Manners and Etiquette

What is a Lady?

A lady is a woman who is revered for her polite behavior and refinement. She is the counterpart of a gentleman. She knows how to behave and speak at all times. Are you a lady? Refinement is attained through good manners, which are rules that set a standard for human behavior. Like showing respect for others, being kind, polite and considerate. Every woman, regardless of her profession or calling in life should be educated and taught the importance of good manners and proper etiquette, which go hand in hand.

Etiquette is about using your manners (behaviors) so that you are comfortable with yourself and, as a result, you are able to make those around you feel comfortable as well. It's about knowing the rules and knowing when it's okay to break them so as to not humiliate others. When you are gracious, thoughtful and kind, other people are attracted to you.

Have you ever seen a woman whose appearance was extremely pleasing to behold? She was fabulously dressed and very beautiful. That is, until she opened her mouth to speak, at which time you discovered her words were incongruent with her visual appearance, and her manners were even worse.

Your manners should match the way you dress and the way you'd like others to know you. I can't count the times I've witnessed beautiful women of all ages who've lost their manners, or perhaps they never acquired them in the first place. What about a beautifully dressed woman in feminine attire who walks, sits and speaks like an unrefined man? In many instances, these women just don't know they are behaving inappropriately or projecting a "split image." They must be taken aside in a gentle, loving and motherly way and educated. Just as Aunt Anita and her girlfriends took me aside and trained me... I must pass it on, femininely and authentically. You must pass it on, too. We are a society who has forgotten that young girls must be trained when it comes to the finer points in life and how to be a lady. It is not only the responsibility of the mother to teach little girls how to become ladies... it is the responsibility of every woman who calls herself a lady. If it is not being demonstrated at home, or for whatever reason many girls aren't getting proper training, then we must all take it upon ourselves to provide the proper training and resources to help form these girls into young ladies. Oh, my... who and where in the world would I be if Aunt Anita had not chosen to participate in my becoming a lady?

Ask yourself these questions:

1.Who is forming our girls?

2.How are they behaving and looking?

3.What do they think of themselves?

What Are The Alternatives?

I've noticed that when we dress sloppily, we speak and act sloppily too—without regard to how others may feel. My goal for myself and for you is that we begin to influence young girls and others for the better by demonstrating good manners and proper etiquette as though it were our next breath. Let's share.

Becoming a Lady

I remember the summer before my senior year of high school, when Aunt Anita and her friends began my training to become a lady. Looking back, it was the beginning of me becoming who I had longed to be, but I had never had the proper language or means to express it. Following my mother's death when I was thirteen, my siblings and I lived with my grandmother. I was the best little girl in the whole wide world… that is, until I turned fifteen. That's when all hell broke loose. Aunt Anita saved me from making a complete fool of myself and ruining my life by coming to get me at sixteen. She took me to live with her, my uncle and two cousins. You see, I felt worthless after my mother's death and believed no one really cared about me—other than saying, "oh, that poor little girl."

But girlfriend, was I ever wrong. I had an aunt who loved me and saw that there was something special in me. She believed I was worthy to be saved and polished. That's when she began her quest to form me. Upon my arrival, I was told we would go shopping the very next day, since I only had one brown paper bag of clothing that was worth anything. I couldn't believe my luck when I saw the beautiful new outfits Aunt Anita bought me that day. For the next several months, each weekend we were in department stores and fabric stores. Everything my aunt couldn't find to fit me properly she made herself—fabulous outfits. Every Saturday I was given a report of how I was progressing. After about four months of dear Auntie training, me and Angela, my cousin, schooling me from her perspective, Aunt Anita commissioned her friends to give me what they had for me. Mrs. Christine Ratcliff pressed my hair, scrubbed my knees and kept me in line with certain crazy *looks*. Dr. Jemma Beckley taught me how to sit and have *proper* conversations by answering certain questions and instructed me on how to ask appropriate questions. Her husband, Dr. David Beckley, took photographs of me and sent them to the Ebony Fashion Fair to get me noticed as a model. I was turned down but my community sure believed in me. It took my Aunt Anita and her friends over a year to get me ready, and when they finished, I was poised and ready to go off to college with confidence and the knowledge of what it means to be a lady. I had the proper tools to maintain what they taught me—self-love, and a new set of electric rollers.

Dining Etiquette

By the time I arrived in Milan, Italy, to pursue the ultimate catwalk, I thought of myself as being a lady—polished and refined. Paul Butler, my San Francisco agent, had picked up and taken over where Aunt Anita left off. What he taught me was like going to graduate school for confidence, self-esteem and fashion. I passed, but it was indeed a trying time for me. Mississippi's refinement did not meet the standards of San Francisco's international urbanity and sophistication. It took several months to a year for me to prepare myself—to get ready for the city; and to *be ready* at the whim of an agent's phone call. Likewise, it took several months for me to feel comfortable with myself in Milan. I was a lady, that was for sure, but my knowledge of proper dining etiquette was put to the test. I didn't know the rules.

Dining in Italy happens every day, twice a day, and it is taken very seriously.

Without proper table manners it's difficult to make a favorable impression during meals. Poor table manners can sometimes be downright embarrassing, for you and others. That's why it's important to know the rules, from the most formal settings to casual outings.

I found myself looking very silly and feeling hungry all the time upon my arrival in Milan, and that first week of my first international excursion. You see, after painstakingly ordering my meal and waiting for its arrival, I was never allowed to finish it. It was my non-verbal communication that the waiters observed. They watched my table manners and, based on what I did with my utensils, they responded.

What I did wrong.

I placed my knife and fork down in the *closed position*, indicating that I was finished.

- By laying my knife and fork diagonally across my plate (not the *resting position—your silverware is placed at the top of your plate)* I indicated to the waiters that I was finished, and my unfinished meal would be taken away.
- I was too embarrassed to say, "Hey, wait a minute, I'm not done here," so I left hungry. That is, until another seasoned model told me, "Chloé, they're very formal here… the waiters are watching you and assuming you know the rules."

Start To Finish Dining Rules for Casual, Semi-Formal and Formal Meals

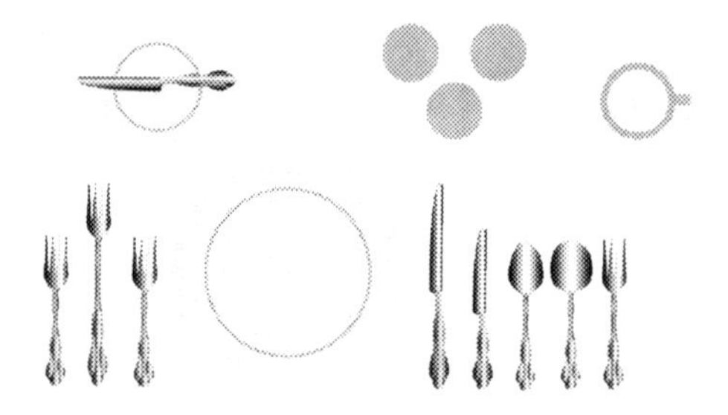

If you remember these quick tips, you'll never be caught off-guard at formal events. Then learn how to live life fabulously by entertaining others and hosting your own dinner parties.

Tips for a semi-formal dinner party:

1.The meal begins when the host unfolds her napkin.

- **a.**Place your napkin in your lap—unfolded if it's a luncheon napkin or in half, lengthwise if it's a dinner napkin.
- **b.**The napkin stays on your lap throughout the entire meal.
- **c.**If you must leave the table before the meal is finished place your napkin in your chair to indicate you will return.

2.Salad Fork—is placed to the far left of the dinner plate.

3.Dinner Fork—is placed to the right of the salad fork.

4.Dessert Fork—is placed to the right of dinner fork and next to the plate.

5.Bread and Butter Plate, with Spreader—is placed above the forks, at the tip of the dinner fork.

6.Dinner Charger—a large plate that adds formal elegance to the table setting is placed right in front of you. *Not intended to be used as a* *plate, it stays on the table throughout the meal and comes off when the dinner plate is taken away.*

7. Dinner Plate—a smaller plate is placed right on top of the charger. *Tip: liquids go to the right of the dinner plate and solids to the left.*

8. Salad knife—is placed to the right of the dinner plate with the serrated edge pointing toward the plate.

9. Dinner Knife—is placed to the right of the salad knife with the serrated edge pointing toward the salad knife.

10. Teaspoon—is to the right of the dinner knife.

11. Soup Spoon—is to the right of the teaspoon.

12. Cocktail Fork—is placed to the right of the soup spoon.

13. Water Glass—is placed above the tip of the blade of the dinner knife.

14. Red Wine Glass—is placed to the right of the water glass.

15. White Wine Glass—is placed to the right of the red wine glass.

16. Coffee Cup—is placed to the right of the white wine glass. *Typically brought out at the end of the meal when coffee is served.*

17. Silverware Tips—always use the silverware that is farthest from your plate—you'll work your way in from the outside.

18. There are two appropriate ways to use a knife and fork to cut and eat your food.

  a. American Style—is cutting your food by holding the knife in the right hand and the fork in the left hand with the fork tines piercing the food to secure it on the plate. Then you cut a few-bite size pieces, lay your knife across the top edge of your plate with the serrated edge facing in toward you, then you change your fork to your right hand and eat, fork tines facing up.

  b. European or Continental Style—is the same as American style in cutting your food; the difference is your fork remains in

your left hand, tines facing down, and the knife in your right hand. You eat the cut food by picking it up with the fork still in your left hand. Food is also pushed onto the back of the fork, tines facing down.

19. General Tips—the above tips are for a semi-formal dinner party or meal at a nice restaurant or banquet. If your meal is casual and you are not being served certain foods or beverages (red wine or salad) then this cutlery, glasses or china would not be place on the table. Only put out china, silverware and glasses that will be used for the meal. Also, when you are chewing, talking or resting, place your cutlery on your plate in the *resting position*—to indicate that you are not finished.

20. Formal Dining Tips—for the most formal meals:

a.Dessert cutlery is placed at the top of the plate.

b.All possible knives are placed to the right of the plate.

c.Each guest has his or her own salt and pepper.

d.All beverages are brought out at the appropriate time.

e.All glasses (except dessert wine glass and water glass), bread plates and salt-and-pepper shakers will be taken away before the dessert is served.

21. Final Tips—when you are finished eating a meal, lay your knife and fork down (in the *closed position*) side-by-side, diagonally across your plate. Serrated edges facing inward and fork tines down, to the left of the knife. Never push your plate away: leave it where it is. Just before you leave the table, place the napkin—unfolded, but not bunched up—to the right of your plate.

22. Money Tip—Break bread, never cut it, and place butter only on the bite-size broken piece.

Step Four—Grooming and Cosmetics

Beholding a well-groomed individual is quite pleasing to my spirit. My eyes begin to twinkle and sparkle and my lips curl upward, leaving me with a little burst of positive energy. Do you know that the measure of a well-groomed woman starts with how good her skin looks? Also, how good her skin looks goes beyond its surface. It's true—how good your skin looks is an *inner beauty being* thing.

How are you being—on the inside?

Having worked in the image, beauty and fashion industries all of my adult life, I've witnessed a lot of vanity… with me right there in the middle. But, what's important and lasting is *Inner Beauty Being*; which always begins with you loving, liking and respecting yourself first. The women who practice inner beauty being are *IBBers—their beauty radiates from the inside out.* They eat the proper foods; which are fueled by chemical substances called essential nutrients, such as: carbohydrates, fats, proteins, minerals, vitamins and water—these nutrients come from the proper and right food sources. So, eating right will help you to reproduce, build, and repair body tissue and to regenerate new skin cells—and we love that.

Water is the most important essential nutrient. It's an elixir within itself—the fountain of youth. Every cell in your body needs water for optimal health, including your skin cells. You could survive for weeks, perhaps even months, without food but you could only last about eight to ten days without water.

Water circulates through your blood transporting oxygen and nutrients to your cells. It helps to maintain the body's natural balance. It has no caloric value, though, and it is not a source of energy within itself. On the other hand, water promotes good digestion and it helps you to absorb the right nutrients from the foods that you eat. It removes your body's waste through urine and sweat and it eliminates digestive waste. It's so good for you!

Your body is made up of about ninety-five percent water and on most days you'll need to drink at least eight to ten cups of water to replenish what you've lost during the day. Water can be replenished also by drinking decaffeinated and non-alcoholic liquids and by eating fresh fruits and vegetables. Getting your fair share of water will cleanse and flush out impurities that clog your pores and diminish your natural beauty. It will help to promote a more supple and youthful complexion. Next time you're dying of thirst, quench it with water.

IBBers believe in herbs and supplements and know that they are essential to their well-being and longevity. They participate in fun, natural and exhilarating activities that encourage them to breathe deeply, giving their body a good cardiovascular workout while rejuvenating their spirit. The breathing that comes from moving your body through fun physical activities is deep, simple, smooth, and strong. This type of breathing will help you to feel more youthful and energetic while at the same time helping you to relax and focus. It will build your heart muscle and clear the clutter from your mind and spirit.

IBBers laugh a lot too—for the fun of it and for the health benefits derived from a good belly laugh. According to Proverbs 17:22, "A joyful heart is the health of the body." Take the time to have fun and laugh. It is not a luxury, like so many of us believe, but just what the doctor ordered. If you're sick, it might make you well. If you're sad it might make you happy. Go on, girl, try it out loud… laugh!

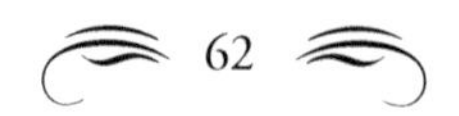

IBBers also know the intrinsic value of friendships with other IBBers and living their lives full out, regardless of where they live, how much money they earn, or whether married or single. They love being with other people *and* being alone. And most importantly, IBBers honor the essence of who they are through quiet time, inner reflection and meditation—a sure and proven way to rejuvenate your body, mind and spirit. Daily meditation can help you get rid of toxins and clear the cobwebs that may have entered your essence, trying to block your natural flow. Meditation will encourage you to relax and to release, allowing you to hear the soft whispered words that are just for you. Consider this: the next time you're *getting ready* think about the selfing process and its grooming layer to see how you're doing with your inner health.

Okay, you now know that the foundation of grooming begins with good skin and a glowing complexion—which is a direct reflection of your inner health and well-being. You also know that paying attention to what goes into your mouth and what's inside your body is key. No amount of topical creams, ointments and serums can be effective when you're covering up for years of neglect.

Exercise, water and meditation, mixed gently and consistently with self-confidence, creates the elixir of life—the fountain of youth!

In order to fully comprehend how to take care of your complexion topically, it's important for you to understand a little more about skin in general—its layers and the types of skin.

Three layers of skin.

The Epidermis is the first and outer layer of your skin—where the dead and dying cells flake off continuously. The good news is that new cells are constantly replacing these old cells. It takes about twenty-eight to thirty days for new cells to regenerate.

The Dermis is the second layer of your skin—it contains blood vessels, hair follicles, nerves, elastic fibers and two essential glands:

- *The oil glands*; which secrete sebum/oil.
- *The sweat glands*; which secrete water and salt. These two glands work together to protect the skin, helping keep the acid balance (pH) of the skin.

The Subcutaneous—Fatty Layer is the third, innermost layer of your skin—it gives firmness to skin and serves as a shock absorber, cushioning against blows and insulating against loss of body heat. Many people only think of the face when they think of skin care. But your skin covers your entire body—from head to toe. Take care of it all!

Basic types of skin

In understanding your particular skin type you will know what skin-care régime will work best for you and how to take care of your beautiful complexion sufficiently.

Take the skin test: Cleanse your face with the products you've been using. Wait a few minutes; then sit comfortably in front of a mirror with good lighting. Ask yourself these questions and record your answers.

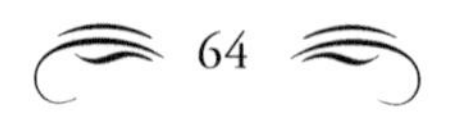

1. How does my complexion look?
2. How does my skin feel?
3. Does it feel tight?
4. Does it feel dry?
5. Does it feel tired?
6. Do I have an oily shine on my forehead and nose?
7. Do I have red blotches?

Now that you have your recorded data, I'd like you to measure it next to the different skin types listed below. If this is too confusing or you don't feel like being bothered, take your data to a consultant at a make-up counter in a nice department store or to a good aesthetician. Being aware of your skin type and needs will empower you and you'll make fewer mistakes when buying new products.

If this still seems intimidating then treat yourself to a facial at an upscale beauty salon or at a medical spa. A licensed aesthetician will be able to give you more insight into your complexion and its needs. And trust me, it's such a nice relaxing treat—you'll love it. I recommend a minimum of six facials per year for normal skin and about eight per year for oily skin.

Normal skin is the type that would be ideal—it appears smooth, supple and soft with very clear pores.

Dry skin feels very thin and delicate, showing very few pores at all. It feels parched and stretched across the bones. If neglected, the tiny lines that appear will turn into full-blown wrinkles.

Oily skin is often shiny with grease and looks thick and coarse. It is prone to enlarged pores and blackheads. Don't panic if you have this skin type. With proper care it can be managed. The good news is that oily skin is the slower skin type to age and wrinkles seem much less obvious.

Do change your pillowcase every night if you have *very* oily skin. The oils and bacteria can build up, re-infecting your skin the next night.

Sensitive skin is normally very finely textured, prone to reddish veins and patches. A light consistency cleanser, moisturizing and a soothing toner are recommended.

Combination skin is a mixture of two or more types of skin. For example, you could be oily in the T-zone (around the nose and forehead) and dry around your eyes or cheekbones—there are several combinations of skin types.

A Total Skin Care Régime

Now that you understand the three layers of skin and types of skin, let's design a total skin care régime that will take you way into your golden years. First and foremost, soap and water will not cut it. Yes, you'll be squeaky clean, but most brands of soaps will strip your complexion of its natural oils and moisture, putting nothing back of value.

Effective Cleansing is the first step. It removes daily oils, dirt and grime that sticks to your skin, clogging your pores. Cleanse your face morning and night with a cleanser that is right for your particular skin type. Different brands of cleansers refer to the same products differently, but usually there is a gentle foaming cleanser that can be used for all

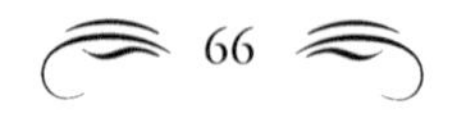

skin types. There is a rich and creamy cleanser for normal to dry skin. There are gel cleansers that are oil free and mild for normal to oily skin and, there are cleansers for very sensitive skin as well. Remember this: If you are not sure of your skin type ask an aesthetician, dermatologist or a consultant at a make-up counter.

Do remember that it is a good idea to cleanse and dry your face with white towels. The dyes in colored towels can irritate your skin.

Do keep your hands off your face throughout the day. They can become dirty and grimy. When you place your hands on your face, you're depositing this dirt and grime right onto your skin.

Exfoliation and facial scrubs gently slough off dead surface cells, allowing your skin to breathe; which actually smoothes and evens the skin's surface. All skin types need exfoliation, some more often than others. When you need a rebalancing boost—exfoliate. Also, for a fabulously smooth feeling all over, take your scrubs into the shower with you at least once a week to get rid of dead skin from the epidermis layer all over. It will allow your newly generated skin to emerge faster, giving the entire body a natural and healthy glow. Girlfriend, you won't be able to keep your hands off yourself.

Toning helps to calm your skin and close your pores after steaming, cleansing and exfoliation. It then prepares it for optimal absorption.

Moisturizing replaces necessary oils and creates a seal over your skin while smoothing and preparing it for make-up. It also protects the skin from the elements. There are oil-free moisturizers that control oil and breakthrough shine as it hydrates. There are rich, hydrating face creams that are wonderful for normal to dry skin.

Do remember to always use appropriate creams, lotions, and facial products for your particular skin type.

Do protect your skin from harmful rays by using sunscreen. As much as eighty percent of wrinkling, age spots and sagging of skin comes from overexposure to the sun. If you have oily skin, stick with water-based sunscreens and try an oil-absorbing gel.

Eye Care is essential because the eye area is very delicate and needs special care. You will need a lightweight and non-greasy cream or gel to condition and renew eye-area skin. I began using eye cream around age twenty-five.

Do remember that under-eye skin is very delicate, so never pull or tug. Instead, delicately pat with your ring finger.

Lip Care keeps lips from cracking and drying. Exfoliate your lips before going to bed by applying a menthol based lip balm—cracked and dry lips can be very unattractive. Upon awakening, gently brush lips with a soft toothbrush or use your wash cloth to gently exfoliate for youthful looking lips all the time.

Nourish and Condition your skin by drinking plenty of water; eating fresh, live foods; getting proper rest and exercise; and by feeding your skin topically with Vitamins A, C and E. Try using a topical C in the morning. Use a topical A at night, then apply glycolic acid on top of the Vitamin A and C. Also, remember that your face also includes your neck and chest area, but *not* your breasts.

Don't smoke. It is horrible for your skin and the nicotine in tobacco narrows blood vessels and prevents oxygen and nutrients from reaching the skin. Also, the act of smoking itself causes skin wrinkles around your mouth and gives you bad breath.

When it Comes to Grooming

Did you know that your hands and fingernails are a big part of your appearance and that you're judged by your "hand-appeal?" That's right, you're judged by how soft your hands are and how nice your nails look. Indeed, manicures and pedicures should be an important part of your skin care and grooming régime. When you shake someone's hand, you'll want that person to focus on you, not on how rough and ragged your hands and nails are.

First, you'll want to keep your hands clean by always washing vigorously after using the bathroom and throughout the day. Always apply a good hand cream to moisturize your hands and cuticles after washing so they don't dry out and crack—and if you want to keep young-looking hands, don't forget to apply sun block to the back of your hands when you know you're going to be outside for extended periods of time. If you neglect your hands, darling, they will certainly defy you and tell your age... maybe even add a few years.

For the life of me, I can never go through to completion with my in-home manicures and pedicures unless I'm using only clear polish. With color, my nails usually end up looking much worse after I'm done with them, but I don't really care. It's a great excuse for me to take advantage of all the pampering I receive from Linda at my favorite nail salon. I usually get a manicure every ten days to two weeks and a pedicure every four to five weeks (you may require more often or less, depending on how fast your nails grow and how well you maintain your polish). Even though I do not maintain my nail polish at home, I do keep my hands and feet moisturized and exfoliated between visits with the right products and tools purchased from my neighborhood beauty supply store.

Do gently push your cuticles back using your towel or an orange stick after bathing or taking a shower.

Do treat yourself to massages—they help to eliminate the negative effects of stress in your life by relaxing your muscles, which in turn relaxes your body and mind.

"The perfectly groomed brow can change your face."
—Kevin Aucoin

Designer Eyebrows

Look at your eyebrows, darling. What do you see? Your brows are like the frame of a beautiful painting, helping to balance your face while showing off the real master-piece—*you*!

Acquiring designer eyebrows may be a little intimidating at first, but once you've gotten in the habit of being well groomed from head to toe, you'll feel incomplete without perfectly groomed brows; especially after you see how designer brows can take years off your appearance and help you to feel absolutely wonderful about yourself. Getting your eyebrows professionally designed is like a mini make-over. Unless you're already a pro at grooming your brows I would suggest letting a professional manage them for you. Then, once you've got the shape you can follow it at home until your next visit.

***

Penciled, stenciled, threaded and waxed, plucked, shaved, trimmed and powdered. Yeah, well, okay, I know, but, they say no pain no gain—right? But, think about it. There is something mysteriously wrong with a unibrow. Besides, with just a little removal of unwanted hair, some filling in of sparse areas or shading a blond brow you can have that gorgeous face of yours framed the way it should be. Fabulously! Since there are several options for maintaining well-groomed brows I feel confident that one of the following techniques or a combination of the following could work well for you and your image maintenance program.

Pencil Enhancement is generally used to fill in thin or sparse areas using short, slanted hair-like strokes with a very sharp brow pencil. Penciled brows may get oily throughout the day and slide right off your face. If you prefer pencils, make sure you choose the right one.

Stencil Enhancement is literally stenciling your eyebrows onto your face by pressing a brow shaped stencil over your brow bone and lightly brushing brow powder over the stenciled area.

Threading is using one hundred percent twisted and rolled cotton thread to lift facial hair from follicles. It's not that painful and only takes about five minutes.

Waxing is spreading a thin layer of very warm wax to the skin, then a cloth or paper strip is pressed on top and ripped off very quickly to remove the unwanted hair, leaving the skin very smooth—if done appropriately. New hair growth is soft and fine—and after repeated waxing some hairs never grow back.

Tweezing is synonymous with plucking and is considered to be the most precise and effective way to shape your brows. It is literally plucking hairs out one by one in the direction in which the brows grow with special tweezers.

Shaving is using a razor to groom the brows or to completely remove the brows (an out-dated look that can age you). New hair growth in shaved area grows back sharp, coarse and messy. A slip of the hand and there goes an eye.

Trimming is snipping too-long brow hairs one at a time with a very small pair of scissors for a well-groomed look.

Powdering is filling in overly plucked and sparse eyebrows using an angled brush and brow powder.

Coloring is simply dying your eyebrows. As fashionable women, we like to change our hair color, and in doing so we must also consider the color of our brows. Choose a shade for your brows that flatters your skin tone and your new hair color.

Tattooing is using tiny needles to inject permanent make-up made of vegetable products into the brow area. This is a wonderful option for women suffering from alopecia and those of us who have completely overplucked our brows. Tattooing also works well if you have gaps or scarring and for women who are just tired of applying brows daily. The hair-stroke method looks natural while the solid method looks dramatic.

The shape of brows to come may change, but the basics of eyebrow grooming will remain the same. However, for extensive re-shaping of the brows, consult a professional and plan on a maintenance program. It's worth it.

Do remember to trim long nose hairs as well.

Let's Make It Up

The foundation to real beauty starts with a healthy lifestyle, which normally produces good skin and a glowing complexion. I've outlined in the previous section how to acquire a show stopping glow from the inside out. Now, let's spotlight your best facial features with the right cosmetics.

"Make-up—oh no... I like natural beauty!" I hear this comment sometimes as I discuss the necessary steps in enhancing a client's image and how cosmetics will play a role. Some of my clients and women in general, like what they call *natural beauty* (they don't wear make-up) because they have never been taught how to apply beautiful, yet simple and natural make-up. I don't know many women who set out to look *unnatural* as a result of their make-up application; although many have, and do. Beautiful women have used make-up since 4000 BC in ancient Egypt, and perhaps even before that. Listen, we all want to look our best, which equates to youthfulness. That's what make-up does—if applied appropriately, it's supposed to simulate youth and good health. A perfect foundation will even out your complexion and flaws, giving the impression of health and youth.

By the end of my freshman year of college, I became so completely off balance with my diet and sleeping that my beautiful complexion turned into an embarrassing mess. As a result of clogged pores and breakouts, my face was filled with acne scars; the result of eating all the wrong foods, minimal water intake and inappropriate cleansing. Aunt Anita took me to a department store make-up counter where she purchased my first set of skin care products, the stat of my skin care régime. I felt good about my new direction, "But still, look at my face," I complained to my aunt. The scars were very visible and quite distressing to me.

"Let me show you how to make your skin look flawless, while it heals," the salesperson said as she placed several products on the counter.

"You're saying you can cover this?" I asked, pointing to a particular area that I had considered covering with a band-aid to conceal my shame. She did not respond, but began applying a sheer liquid foundation to the scarred and discolored areas of my face with a sponge applicator. She performed a couple of other tricks, then handed me a mirror.

"It's like a miracle," I laughed, not believing my own eyes. My complexion had the appearance of flawlessness. My self-esteem increased immediately. You see, Aunt Anita cared enough to introduce me to proper skin care and a few simple make-up tips that helped to transform the way I viewed myself at the time. That was the beginning of my *on-purpose self-love* and of taking care of myself— from the inside out. This was the beginning of me becoming an inner beauty being.

Beauty matters, darling!
Women have chased beauty and youthfulness since ancient Egyptian times.

Beauty matters… significantly, especially when it comes to mating and reproductive success. What a particular man wants in a woman stacks up differently from what a woman wants in a man. On a scale of one to five, men say that attractiveness is number one on their list, followed by commitment, social skills, resources and then sexiness. For women, though, commitment is number one, followed by social skills, resources and attractiveness, with sexiness bringing up the rear. These aren't new preferences for either of the sexes. Rather, they have evolved over millennia.

So, my dear lady friend, if you're married, it seems like a pretty good idea to take good care of yourself for increased well-being and happiness. You'll feel so much better about yourself in all areas of your life. And then, I strongly encourage you to look especially delicious for your husband. Men want their wives or significant others to look good for them, and not just every now and then, either. Listen, and just roll with me for a minute. I know that this might be a sensitive area, but we've got to be realistic about this topic and get through it, together. Generally speaking, men are visual, so appearance is at the top of their list when it comes to choosing a mate. I'm willing to bet that when you and your husband were dating you went out of your way to look good for him—right? He probably pursued or chased you and the two of you participated in activities together that you considered romantic, fun and exhilarating, or you went along with it to please him. This was probably thrilling for him, and no doubt, he thought you were beautiful, fine, sexy, and, of course, all the other dynamic and fabulous traits that he adores about you. But, remember like most men he's probably visual, which means appearance is at the top of his list. Okay, so it's the beautiful, fine, sexy side of you that I've been commissioned to talk about on behalf of husbands.

A man wants his woman to be well groomed, to take care of herself physically, as well as emotionally and spiritually, and to look good around him. Now, I'm not talking about being skinny or fat here. What I am talking about is working toward being your personal best. Some men say they feel let down, or even robbed when the woman they love lets herself go and does nothing about it.

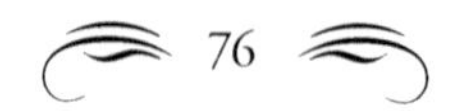

According to Shaunti Feldhahn's research for her book, *For Women Only—What You Need To Know About The Inner Lives Of Men*, your man may feel unvalued and unhappy when you don't take care of yourself. I love this little book and actually learned a lot about my husband, my son, and men in general. The following are excerpted comments from two men in Shaunti's book.

"Shaunti, those women need to realize that their doubling in size is like a man going from being a corporate raider to a minimum-wage slacker—and assuming it has no effect on his spouse. A woman's appearance is a simple yet important part of happiness in a marriage…"

"We need to see that you care about keeping our attention on you—and off other women. Sometimes it is so hard for us to look away. It takes a lot of work and a lot of effort. But it helps me so much if I see that my wife is willing to do her part and purposefully work toward staying in shape and looking good."

If you're single and would like to become married one day, I would highly suggest that you pay close attention to yourself in regard to grooming and attractiveness as well. For those of you who are single and loving it, I hear you. But let me suggest that you pay close attention to attractiveness, too, which deposits magnificent gold nuggets into your self-worth account, and your bank account, too. The bottom line—the way you look matters everywhere. First it matters at home, and just as importantly, it matters at work, at the gym, your children's school and at the super market. Do you see where I'm going with this? I will outline how you can perfect your authentic image from head to toe without feeling stripped of your already limited time. And once you have it down, you'll love it and wonder what took you so long.

Make-Up Essentials

The tricks to applying simple yet gorgeous make-up lie within your technique and your tools. When you have the right tools and know how to use them correctly you'll have more fun and acquire the look that you're going for. First, you'll need special applicators and a collection of good brushes, which can be purchased separately or in less expensive kits at beauty supply stores.

I learned how to apply basic make-up (lip-stick and mascara) in high school and, of course, loving everything about fashion, image, make-up and style as a teenager, I began to experiment more in college after adding new products purchased to conceal my acne scars. But, once I got back home, I really didn't understand how to apply my new cosmetics the right way. Although I'd have to admit I did better than most of the girls in my dormitory. When I moved to San Francisco, however, and became a fashion model, it was Paul Butler, my new agent, who took me under his wing, taking over where Aunt Anita left off.

Paul took me to Neiman Marcus in Union Square. "I want you to get used to using the best of everything," he said calmly as he sat down beside me at the make-up counter. It was fascinating watching Paul as he instructed the saleslady in what he called "the appropriate tools and cosmetics for Chloé." At the time, I felt special and believed these particular tools were just for me; but soon I learned that all models had the same tools in their make-up cases. Again, the tricks to applying simple, yet gorgeous make-up come from your technique *and* the appropriate tools. Following is the list of tools that I purchased that day and have continued to replace throughout the years.*

•**A** Large Powder Brush
•**A** Blush Brush
•**A** Contour Brush
•**A** large Fluff Brush
•**A** Small Fluff Brush
•**A** Flat Concealer Brush
•**A** Flat, Stiff, Angled Brow Brush
•**A** Brow Groomer
•**A** Metal Lash Comb
•**A** Retractable Lip Brush
•**A** Small, Flat, Angled Eyeliner Brush
•**S**ponge Eye Shadow Applicators
•**L**atex Wedges
•**C**otton Swabs
•**C**osmetic Powder Puff
**Always keep your make-up brushes clean.*

You would be surprised by the number of women who do not keep their make-up brushes clean. Please, understand that your cosmetic tools and brushes harbor lots of oils, bacteria and dirt, which deposits right onto your face and into your pores, if your tools aren't clean.

Cleaning your brushes should be an integral part of your healthy skin care maintenance program. Synthetic hair brushes are okay and less expensive, but I like the real deal—natural hair bristles—for my cosmetic brushes. They just feel better on my skin and they're easier to clean and dry.

I have used eye make-up remover to clean my brushes, as well as face wash, antibacterial soap or shampoo, which have all worked well. However, personally I prefer to use my face wash, since my brushes are touching my face.*

Cleaning Your Cosmetic Brushes

1. First, never leave your brushes soaking in water if the handles are wood. This will destroy them.
2. Gather all the brushes that you intend to clean.
3. Run warm water over the bristles of the brush.
4. I usually pour a small amount of my face wash into the palm of my hand and saturate the wet bristles into the face wash and work into a foamy lather.
5. Rinse and repeat until the running water turns clear.
6. Air dry; or if your bristles are natural hair you may blow dry your brushes on low heat.

Tip: *You may also purchase a specialized cleaning solution to clean your brushes from your neighborhood beauty supply store.*

"I only have to do three things to look halfway decent: curl my eyelashes, fill in my eyebrows and put some lipstick on."
—Courteney Cox

Here is my take on looking "halfway decent." If I were allowed to have only two cosmetic products in my make-up case, they would be the *right* brown pencil that could be used as an eyeliner and for filling in my brows, for lining and filling in lips, and maybe for a little color on my cheeks. Then I'd use black mascara to darken and thicken my lashes, making my eyes "pop," giving me a more youthful look.

What about you? What are your two to three tricks you could use to look halfway decent with minimum time and limited cosmetic products? Before you begin your make-up application, you'll want to start out with a clean canvas—so cleanse thoroughly and moisturize your face. Then follow these simple steps.

Beautiful Make-Up—Three Techniques

Fast, Natural and Pretty Make-up

This is your "no make-up" *look*—the look that you wear to the supermarket, the gym, car pooling the kids, and other everyday activities. You'll need five products (foundation, blush, loose powder, mascara and a lip color) for this particular look.

Step 1: Foundation

Apply a light layer of your foundation, making sure to blend at all edges. Applied correctly, it will even out your complexion and give you a more youthful look. The color of your foundation should match your skin. Test the color on your jawline and wait a few minutes to see if it matches your complexion before buying. *When I am short of time and only need minor coverage, I apply my foundation with my fingers just in the places I need it.*

Step 2: Blush

A little blush is probably necessary, so make sure you use the appropriate medium-size blush brush, one that fits the size of the apples of your cheeks when you smile. Too much blush and you'll run the risk of looking clownish. So, the first trick is to tap the blush

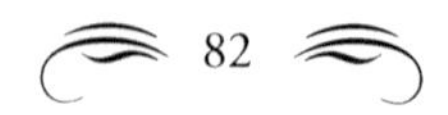

brush very lightly with the tips of the bristles into the blush—you'll want to avoid picking up too much color. Next, blow or tap the brush a couple of times to remove excess blush. Remember to smile, then tap across cheeks. Don't blend out too much toward the hairline; otherwise you'll look like you're stuck in the eighties.

Step 3: Loose Powder

Use your large powder brush now (without excess powder on it) to blend by sweeping the brush over your entire face to get a natural and pretty look.

Step 4: Mascara

Mascara is so fabulous! It makes every woman look good; a little or a lot, if applied correctly, will enhance your eyes by making your lashes appear darker and thicker. Your eyes will appear larger—a sign of youth. Gel-based mascara can enhance your lashes, giving you a beautiful natural effect. With this "no make-up" look—I usually suggest that you skip the mascara on the bottom. However, if this just isn't you, then apply mascara to bottom lashes first, by holding the wand in a vertical manner and stroking once or twice; then wait for them to dry. Next, tilt chin up a little, look out and slightly down, then apply mascara to top lashes by placing wand very close to topside of lashes and brush downward. Now, brush your lashes up with the mascara wand to lift and separate. Or you may use a lash comb to lift and separate and to also remove excess mascara.

Step 5: Lipstick

To have your very own signature lip color says a lot about a woman. You'll want one for this natural, pretty look as well as for your other two looks. But, first, you'll want to have smooth, kissable lips that don't scratch—so always apply a little lip balm before going to bed or before you apply your lipstick. I like cream and matte lipsticks for day time; they have staying power. Save your gloss for evening and night. Choose your everyday color based on your natural lip shade. Now, glide your pretty lipstick over your lips, blot to remove excess color. Glide lipstick on again and blot again to even out the texture. This should last for several hours.

If you follow these simple techniques, you'll never be caught without a pretty glow that looks completely natural while boosting your self-esteem.

"I love the confidence that makeup gives me."
—Tyra Banks

You don't have to be a super-model to know that make-up can help build your confidence. It helps you to project a poised, polished and professional look.

Poised, Polished and Professional Make-up

Step 1: Foundation

Apply a light layer of your foundation, making sure to blend at all edges. This is the time to use a sponge applicator. When I am seriously seeking a fabulous look, I apply my foundation with a sponge for more coverage and control, as opposed to using my fingers, which I do for the natural and pretty technique.

Step 2: Concealer

If *necessary*, dot concealer around nose, under eyes and on any blemishes or imperfections, and blend. *Don't* overdo under-eye concealer, especially if you have heavy dark circles and bags. Instead, draw attention to upper eyes by using extra coats of mascara. Most importantly, always get enough sleep and rest.

Step 3: Blush

Use the same technique as in Step 2 in *Fast Natural and Pretty Make-up.*

Step 4: Loose Powder

With a large powder brush, apply loose powder. Tap the powder brush very lightly with the tips of the bristles into the loose powder—you'll want to avoid picking up too much. Next, blow or tap the brush a couple of times to remove excess powder. Now, try sweeping the brush over your entire face to softly blend and to set your makeup, giving you a poised, polished and professional look.

Step 5: Eye Shadow

Your eyes are the windows to your soul, the most important feature of your face. If you use eye shadows, make sure to blend well and use them appropriately. A time saver and easy trick for work is to use the same lighter color to highlight the entire eye area, from eyelid to upper lid, leading up to the brow area. Then use a darker color in the fold of the eye for contouring, helping you to achieve a nice almond shape.

Step 6: Eye Liner

For a simple, sophisticated look skip Step 5 and try a black or brown thin line very close to the upper lashes. No shadow is necessary.

Step 7: Mascara

Curl your lashes if necessary and add two coats of mascara. See mascara tips in Step 4 of *Fast, Natural and Pretty Make-up.*

Step 8: Lipstick

As a busy woman, you'll no doubt want your morning lipstick to last at least until after lunch. First, line your lips with a color a shade or two darker than your lipstick. Then shade in the entire lip area with your liner pencil and apply your lipstick. For a super long-lasting and defined look, layer lipstick on top of matching liner, blot several times and reapply lipstick for hours of luscious lips.

"Glamour is innate—you either have it or you don't."
—Pamela Church-Gibson

The right shade of lipstick can take you straight from your day look into instant glamour for the evening. And don't be afraid to add extra coats of mascara, either. *You glow, girl!*

Glamorous and Alluring Make-up

For **Steps 1, 2, 3 and 4:** Follow the *Poised, Polished and Professional* application steps.

Step 5: Eye Shadow

You know the basic techniques. Now you may want to go all out for glamorous eye make-up. First, for long-lasting eye shadow try putting a very thin coat of concealer, foundation or a neutral-colored liquid eye shadow over your eyelid and choose one of these two fabulous looks.

Simple Elegance

- For an easy, elegant look with eye liner—create a heavier line using a narrow sponge tip applicator. Now, smudge slightly with your eye shadow brush for a smoky, romantic look.

The Eyes Have It!

- Using a shadow brush apply a light-colored base powder eye shadow from your lashes to your brow.
- Cover your lower lids with a medium-toned to dark-toned shade.
- If you select a medium-toned shade then you will want to use a darker shade to contour the crease.
- If you select a dark-toned shade for your lids then you'll want to select a medium-toned shade for the crease.
- Blend and blend again with your eye shadow brush or brushes. Be careful not to transfer colors. If you use too much you may tone the colors down by using your loose powder on a sponge applicator or your cosmetic powder puff.

Step 6: Eye Liners

Using *Eye Shadow as Eyeliner*, select a medium to dark shade to line your eyes.

- Use your small, flat-angled eyeliner brush.
- Hold your brush so that the shortest tip is closest to your lash line.
- Begin at the inside of the upper lid and work out toward the outer corner.
- Gently stroke the brush over your eye shadow.
- For a more dramatic look—wet your eyeliner brush before dipping it into your shadow. It will dry quickly.

Using Pencil Eyeliners

- Pencil eyeliners should be adequately sharpened—it gives your eyes soft definition, but smears easily.
- Using a shadow over the pencil can be very long-lasting.

Using Liquid Eyeliners

- If you're going for precision and drama, then liquid eyeliner might be for you. Be patient, though. It might be a little difficult to apply at first, but if you practice, I'll bet you'll have this technique down in no time.
- Don't be heavy-handed.

Using Cake Eyeliners

- Cake eyeliner comes in a pot and can be applied in the same manner as liquid eyeliner.
- Cake eyeliner is creamier than liquid. It can be purchased or made by dipping a wet eyeliner brush into a dark shadow—sweeping gently through your shadow several times.
- Allow liquid and cake liners to dry before opening your eyes completely.

Step 7: Mascara

See basic mascara tips in Step 4 of *Fast, Natural and Pretty Make-up.*

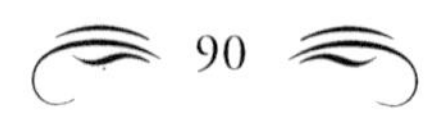

- For bold and glamorous eyes, don't be afraid to add additional, thin coats of mascara.
- Comb lashes with your metal eyelash comb or a disposable plastic wand after they've dried to remove clumps and to acquire a more natural look.
- I love black, but all black mascaras are not true black—some are bluish-gray. Swipe across a white tissue before buying to make sure you're getting black.
- If you cannot bring yourself to skip the mascara from your bottom lashes then please, not too much; one thin layer is fine.

Step 8: Lipstick

Luscious, *Smooth and Sexy Lips* will triumph every time. Beautiful plump lips are a sign of youth and natural beauty. In fact, the most beautiful and kissable look for lips is the one described in the *Fast, Natural and Pretty Make-up* section. Yes, darling, your natural lip shade, spiked with a little gloss, is the most kissable lip look.

*Irresistible Kissable Glamour**

1. Make sure your lips are smooth and soft by massaging a lip balm, like Chapstick (which also helps to keep your lipstick on longer) on your lips and wait a few minutes.
2. Line your lips with a shade the same color as your lips.

3. Use your *Fast, Natural and Pretty* lipstick color or another one that allows your natural lip color to show through (a sheer lipstick or gloss).
4. You may apply your lipstick straight from the tube if you like.
5. Blend well along your natural lip line.
6. Apply your lip gloss with the wand or a lip brush, or you may smooth it out with your fingertip.

** Dark smoky eyes will look fabulous with this lip look.*

Seductive Glamour*

1. Line your lips with a color one shade darker than your lipstick.
2. Shade in the entire lip area with your liner pencil.
3. For a spectacular precise look layer your lipstick on top of matching lip liner with your lip brush.
4. Blot several times with a one-ply tissue or with hair endpapers and reapply lipstick.
5. Apply your lip gloss with a lip brush.
6. Enjoy a super-fabulous and long-lasting defined lip look.

** A thin dark line framing the eye with several coats of mascara would look fabulous with this lip look.*

Lip Tips

- **For fabulously smooth lips all the time**

  1. Moisturize lips nightly with a medicated lip balm.

2.Exfoliate your lips in the morning by gently rubbing with a clean wash cloth.

3.Try pressing a wet tea bag against lips for thirty seconds for sexy soft lips in a few seconds.

•Beautiful Balanced Lips

1.If your lips are too thin, outline your upper and lower lips just outside your natural lip line and fill in with lipstick. Apply lip gloss to the center of your mouth.

2.If your lips are too thick, make sure to apply your foundation to your lips. Then outline your lips just inside the natural lip line and apply lipstick. Avoid too much lip gloss. For electric shine, try a lip lacquer, alone or over lipstick.

Do remember to remove your make-up before going to bed. Your skin sheds and replenishes itself while you sleep, so make sure it's clean.

"The hair is the richest ornament of women"
—Martin Luther

Hair Say

Brittle, broken, burned, colored, dandruff, dry, frizzy, gray, oily, permed, relaxed, slow growing, split ends, thinning... Rarely do I meet a woman who is completely happy with her hair for an extended period of time—unless she has chosen to wear it cut very low, wear natural locks or shave it bald, by choice, and even that may have its challenges.

Your name can't save you from it. Your stylist can't save you, no matter how fabulous he or she may be. Where you live can't save you nor can your hair texture or hair type save you. Trust me, you are guaranteed to have a few bad-hair days, if not many. But, in order to have the upper hand, to be able to minimize these days, the most important thing is to know what you're working with.

What's your hair type in its natural state?
Is it fine, medium or thick?
Is the texture bushy, curly, kinky, wavy or straight?

Knowing your hair type and texture won't completely eliminate problems but this knowledge will certainly give you the upper hand when it comes to making the best decisions about your own tresses—what you can and can't do with your hair *and* to it. Also, this information can guide you in perfecting your authentic image in regard to maintaining your overall appearance so that you can design a nourishing healthy hair régime and know what styles will work best for you.

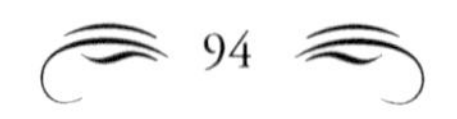

In its natural state, I have fine, bushy/wavy hair… but, right now, I have fine, relaxed, color-treated hair (double chemicals) that needs extra-special care. As a young girl I had gorgeous fluffy hair; Momma shampooed, oiled and pressed it every Saturday morning. Daddy fussed and said, "All she needs on her hair is grease and water."

Momma never burned me and I never lost one strand of hair, other than natural shedding. On the other hand, when I worked as a model, on several occasions my wet hair was pulled out and my dry hair was burned out by stylists prior to fashion shows and photo shoots. For them it was all about *the look*. I've had other stylists relax my hair, leaving it broken, sliding right down the shampoo bowl. I have been a slave to the excessive use of blow dryers, flat irons and curling irons… oh, the things I've put my fine, bushy/wavy hair through!

So, How Can a Girl Win?

A girl can win with good self-esteem, an engaging personality, great skin, a big smile, fabulous shoes and the very best, most fabulous hairstylist you can find.

Hair style is the final tip-off whether or not a woman really knows herself.
—Hubert de Givenchy

First and foremost, you've got to have a stylist who knows you are serious about your hair. They've got to understand that it is *all* about you while at the same time the two of you are in agreement that he/she is definitely *the* most-high fabulous stylist. Your very reason for being there is because you know this. Agreements are powerful.

Now, this is why it is critical that you know your hair type, texture and *hair say*—your hair stories. You want to be able to communicate this and other vital information to the stylist. That's why stylists have consultations first. Get it all out, darling—tell him/her everything. If he/she doesn't want to listen, that stylist is not the right one for you. *Leave!*

Sure, you can get an okay hairdo from beauty schools for a faction of the cost. But the job of the most-high fabulous stylist is to make you look absolutely gorgeous—every visit—otherwise what's the point?

Your Responsibilities in Maintaining Good Hair

1. You've got to do your part by finding the best stylist for you.
2. Know your hair's personality. What happens to it when it's exposed to humidity, rain, heat, perms, relaxers, color, blow drying, hot irons and styling products?
3. Use the best products for your hair's personality.

Your Hair Stylist is Responsible for the following:

1. *The stylist* mus*t* understand your hair say. Most of us have hair stories that we want to share with a new stylist. I must always tell new stylists my hair stories. My hair is very fragile all around the perimeter; this information helps a stylist to make more informed decisions about chemicals applied in that area.

2. *The stylist* needs to talk with you about your hair type and texture.
3. *The stylist* must discuss with you your lifestyle, fashion personality type and hair goals.
4. *The stylist* job is to restore and/or maintain healthy hair.
5. *The stylist* should help you design an in-home maintenance régime that is just right for you.
6. *It's the stylist* job to consistently please you by providing wonderful services and a great haircut and style—every visit.
7. *The stylist* needs to inform you of all hair options, including new cutting-edge products, old reliable and proven products, wigs, weaves and the many types of hair extensions, beauty magazines and hair shows, and anything that he/she believes you would be interested in when it comes to hair and beauty. You want a *progressive* stylist.

With the right hair stylist, the right cut and style, a personal maintenance plan and a little time—sleek, sophisticated and fabulous hair *can* be yours, darling. Remember, you and your stylist have an agreement to make this happen.

Step Five—Clothing and Fashion

What kind of relationship are you having with your clothes? Fashion and clothing have the power to influence you in a profound way. This effect can be positive or negative, and it can have a major impact upon your self-esteem, your mood and the impressions you make on other people. The messages that your clothing convey can profoundly affect the perceptions of others—and they affect you as well. Therefore, it is always to your advantage to dress for effect and to *look the part.* As individuals and professionals, though, we have a collection of self-images to choose from. It is important that we understand that the choice of image at any given time is based on role demands.

Ask yourself:

- **W**ho am I being in the world?
- **W**hat do I want to project or communicate about myself?
- **H**ow do I want others to perceive me?

With these questions answered, you will have a better understanding of the big picture for your life and how you want to advance, which determines your ideal wardrobe and what will work best for you while at the same time what will project your authentic image. When you begin designing, creating and perfecting your authentic image it is necessary to take into account the role you will be playing in your life, as well as your lifestyle.

If you are the vice president of marketing at a Fortune Five Hundred company, your work attire will probably be quite different from a middle-school special education teacher. And no doubt, your lifestyle will probably be different as well. If you are an art dealer you will probably dress differently from an accountant or a radiologist. Even a television news anchor would dress differently from a film editor.

Are you urban, suburban, small town, international or rural? Are you married or single? Do you have children? What is your age? Do you work from home? Do you travel often? Do you entertain friends and family and/or clients and business associates? When you're home, do you like to lounge, cook or garden? My point is—all of these multi-dimensional parts of who you are being, or want to be, must be taken into consideration in order for you to be authentic in the way you are expressing yourself visually. So, then, to make sure that you're ready to *get ready* for all the areas of your life while remaining authenticity—you'll want to give your wardrobe a fresh and energetic workout by:

1. Assessing everything that you have in your closets and drawers.
2. Clearing out everything that is not consistent with your big picture of who you are and where you're headed in your life.

Caution: Unless you're clear about your direction in life, you may find yourself creating a persona that is inauthentic, and in fact, incongruent with your true essence and where you really want to go. Now, listen, if your goal is to create characters for your life then that's fine. Go for it. This can be necessary at times. In fact, some careers even demand various personas. But, if your objective is to create and project a reliable and trustworthy appearance which meets the requirements of any occasion, then let's get serious for a moment.

Ask yourself these questions:

1.What do I want to communicate about myself to the world?

2.How important is my image to my success in *becoming* who I want to be and in *communicating* what I want others to know about me?

Please! Before you take on the task of completing your closet evaluation, auditing your wardrobe and purchasing new pieces to include into your existing wardrobe, I want you to understand the social significance of clothing, and the relationship between fashion and identity. As I have indicated before, people judge you based on how you look and the clothes you wear. Make your clothes work for you, not against you.

One of the first comprehensive studies of the social significance of clothing was conducted in 1950 at Michigan State University. It showed that urban, white-collar workers dressed to impress others, while rural, blue-collar workers were concerned more about durability and performance of clothing. The only thing that has changed today is there are fewer rural, blue-collar workers and millions upon millions of workers from many varied fields of work who realize the importance of dressing for effect and to impress. Most successful people build wardrobes that take them where they want to go in life. With that said, I encourage you to seriously consider the big picture for your life; otherwise your endeavors may feel superficial and staged.

Like many women I know, you probably have clothes in your closet that you haven't worn for years—and there are possibly pieces in your wardrobe that you have not worn at all. Get rid of these clothes, darling. Someone else can really use them and would be very pleased to have them. But, first, I want you to understand why you have these unworn pieces and clothes that misrepresent you hanging in your closet in the first place.

In order to do this, I want to show you how your lifestyle, and your fashion personality type, combined with your body type and shape will give you every advantage to looking absolutely fabulous and appropriate for any and all occasions. Integrating all of these elements into the way you think about your visual appearance helps you to understand what works and what does not work in building your best wardrobe and image.

Lifestyle

Your lifestyle is the way you live your life, darling. It's the ways in which you express yourself; your interest and opinions, your purchasing habits and what you consume. It's what you do in your leisure time, the entertainment and activities that you enjoy. It's the foods you love and enjoy. It's where you live and how you live, it's how you treat your body and the way that you dress it. In other words, your lifestyle reflects your attitudes, views and values.

For the purpose of this book and for making my image enhancement points stand out, I'll mainly refer to lifestyle in terms of the personal and professional roles that you may be playing in your life or aspiring to play in the world. I'll also show how these roles usually reflect themselves through our wardrobes and how we dress. Remember, in many cases, the way you dress is viewed as an extension of your physical self and something that you should pay close attention to. If you stick with me, I'll introduce you to six fabulous women—illustrating through them how to design and create your most fabulous wardrobe.

Fashion Personality Types

Knowing your clothing and fashion personality type can solve many fashion dilemmas and keep you from ending up on the worst dressed list. Also, it will help you to save precious time and energy by keeping you out of stores that are incongruent with your authentic image. Knowing your fashion personality type increases your self-assurance about the clothes you *do* buy.

Are you *Avant Garde, Bohemian, Casual, Classic, Conservative, Country & Western, Dramatic, Flirtatious, Glamorous* or *Rebellious*? In this section I'll describe these ten clothing and fashion personality types and show how most of us are multi-dimensional when it comes to our likes and dislikes about the clothes that we buy and what we actually wear. In most cases we have dominant pieces in our wardrobes that we continue to go back to or rely on. We feel good in these pieces, and family and friends tell us we look good when we're wearing them. This particular clothing type may represent your fashion personality type and bring out the best in you—for reasons I'll point out later when I introduce Madison, Ava, Isabella, Angela, Hannah and Rebecca, six amazing women whom I've grown to admire, love and cheer for. I'll show you how I have assisted each of them to craft an amazing wardrobe based on being a fully balanced woman who loves and respects herself and her body. They are all *Inner Beauty Beings.*

Each of these women loves living life fabulously—which they believe helps them to make the most of themselves and their lives. You'll see how the image and styles created for each woman is based on her body type, her shape and proportions, her fashion personality type, her age, career and lifestyle, but first, let's check out ten different clothing and fashion personality types. See where you find yourself.

Clothing and Fashion Personality Types

Avant Garde is high fashion at its best, or worst, depending on who is wearing it and how. At best it can include chic, one-of-a-kind pieces from your favorite designer's custom-made collections. This clothing style is very expensive and fitted for individual body types and sizes. When you think of Avant Garde think haute couture and high fashion—with designer names attached like Saint Laurent, Valentino, Chanel, de la Renta and the like. Think classic old guards whose image and style were impeccable. Now flash back to middle-aged divas from the 1980's and all of their padded couture. And finally, fast forward to flashy new money socialite divas of today who will drop several thousand dollars for a flashy dress that will be worn once or twice before it's auctioned off for charity.

Bohemian in its true essence is a counter-culture to real fashion, a vagabond, so to speak. Today, however, it is considered an unstructured chic look for those who wish to express themselves in somewhat of an eclectic style by mixing and layering patterns and fabric textures. When you think of bohemian think: ruffled skirts in fabrics like chiffon, velvet and light-weight cottons and Indian-and African-inspired prints. Pair this with long flowing tops in silks, chiffons and lace with jeans. *Don't forget* to accessorize with gorgeous Indian-or African inspired bangles, layers of gold or silver necklaces and belts. How about 1970's inspired boots?

Casual at its best is youthful, easy-going, simple and unpretentious, but with a flair. Casual no longer means wearing your old worn-out clothes around the house or to the gym. Today's casual is more fitted: it can be preppy, or even somewhat sexy in a clean and simple way. If your image and personality type leans toward casual you are more inclined to wear cottons, denim and khaki.

Classic is chic, yet simple and feminine; the designs and styles have a timeless appeal and can be worn year after year without the worry of being "out of fashion." This image and personality type seems to fit in, and even soar in certain environments, especially in the corporate arena. The lines of the classic look are structured yet simple, elegant and exquisitely tailored.

Conservative is modest, reserved, soft and feminine, with a tendency to lean toward simple flowing lines with rounded curves. If this is your image and personality type, you will never run the risk of being called sleazy or sloppy. You may gravitate to traditional old-fashioned girlish features like small prints and lace. Your clothes are never too tight and price is not an issue for you. Your accessories are small to medium and you like gold, diamonds and pearls.

Country & Western evokes feelings of being wild and strong—a woman who can take care of herself. This style represents American values and rugged individualism. You are not afraid of getting a little dirt under your manicured nails and you probably have a few pairs of fabulous cowboy boots in your shoe collection. Even though you may be sporting denim, rhinestones and fringes, comfort is important to you in your selection of durable natural fibers. Cowgirls, celebrities, the general public, and the fashion runways of New York have all gone Western at some point.

Dramatic is bold, confident, striking and chic. You love drama and it spills over into your wardrobe. People often think of you as being glamorous, but be careful not to take it too over the top, or you'll run the risk of being glitzy; which is okay for show business, darling, but not for everyday life. You are not your typical mix and match kind of girl either. You are a risk taker who goes for crisp tailored ensembles with strongly defined shoulders and ornate jewelry. Bold colors set you apart from the crowd and you are often seen in black, which fits your style beautifully.

Flirtatious is feminine and romantic. You love getting attention based on your seductive, girlie side and you're not afraid to tease and entice by wearing easy flowing fabrics that float and wrap around your body. You gravitate to delicate, sexy pieces in fabrics such as cozy, superfine wools and cashmeres, romantic satins and silks, easy flowing jersey, elegant vintage-looking dresses, chiffons and exquisite lace. You are not inclined to purchase baggy, boxy or loose fitting clothes. However, you love to mix and match, creating that "just right" girlie look.

Glamorous is timeless and beautiful. You are confident, resilient, poised, polished and perfectly put together. You know how to look fabulous for any occasion. Being glamorous is a mind set—giving the impression of a tasteful, stylish and high-end lifestyle that spills over into everything that you do. Your wardrobe is uncomplicated, well fitted, and made out of the finest fabrics and materials. You are not trendy. You prefer to build your wardrobe one piece at a time, which includes chic, one-of-a-kind pieces, expensive designer reproductions, special vintage pieces, the right handbags, shoes and accessories and, of course, that oh-so-fabulous perfect black dress. Being glamorous is about quality not quantity.

Rebellious is a feminine maverick who goes for shock appeal—using clothes to make a bold and edgy statement that oozes controversy or sexuality, or both. You're different and you want everyone to know it. For you, there is no good or bad, right or wrong way of dressing or expressing your individuality. For the most part your clothes are of good quality—high-end designer pieces mixed with vintage, thrift, discount or department store items. Your renegade spirit encourages you to create outfits that others would never think of wearing (think of artist like Lil' Kim and Pink). You mix and match distinctive patterns, fabrics and styles, making it difficult for anyone to copy your unique style.

It's nice to have a great female composer in the program and add her color.
—Cecilia Bartoli, Colortura Soprano

Color Power

A woman with style has a good understanding of basic colors with regard to her core wardrobe and how these colors can be mixed with other colors to perfect a positive and powerful non-verbal communication tool called *Color Power.* She knows her best colors; and, she also knows the color her personality adds to the program—in the same magnificent style as that of a coloratura soprano.

You, too, can acquire color power—if you properly exploit the colors that work best for you, and take advantage of them in creating and perfecting your authentic wardrobe and image. Your personal, most fabulous color combinations are waiting to display themselves in your wardrobe, darling—for play, work, evening or any special occasion. Your best colors will complement and enhance your skin tone, hair and eye color. They will make you feel good… and look marvelous. Do take advantage of them.

A color's personality can be energetic and sparkling, with the power to motivate, inspire and attract people to you—another color's personality can be dull, lethargic and boring, possibly pushing people away from you. But, the *right* combination of colors used appropriately can give you super-star, magical style—style that sets you apart in a positive way.

If you already know your best colors, that's fabulous! You already have the upper hand when it comes to coordinating wonderful color combinations for your core wardrobe, which consists of suits, jackets, skirts, pants, blouses and tops, and dresses. However, if you don't know and need a little assistance or a frame of reference as to how colors harmonize, complement or clash, it's as simple as hiring an image consultant to assist you by conducting a personal color analysis, which will help you determine your best colors.

Or, if you'd like to try to determine your best colors for yourself, first, you'll want to find a color wheel to get a visual representation of the reds, yellows and blues, combined with the blacks and whites, and the amazing possibilities of beautiful hues, shades, and tints that are possible. Then, you'll want to determine if you have warm undertones (yellow or golden), which are referred to as *spring or autumn,* or cool undertones (blue or pink), referred to as *summer or winter.* This assessment will provide you with suggestions for colors, shades and tints that can work for you based on your skin tone, hair and eye color. Don't be too rigid, though. Once you know what works I fully expect you to have the confidence to experiment with different combinations.

Having worked in the image and fashion industry for more than twenty-five years, I *do* know that some women can actually wear colors that do not fall into their "color season." These women have enormous confidence. They know just how to mix and match and how to wear a particular shade or tint. They embrace fashion and know what's hot and what's not; however, they are not trendy... they have *style.*

Take a look at the characteristics of the four "color seasons" below and determine which season most accurately matches your traits. If you have cool undertones your basic core colors are white, black, gray, navy and taupe. If you have warm undertones your basic core colors are ivory, brown, camel and beige.

Wardrobe Core Color Basics: black, brown, blue, navy, gray, taupe, camel, ivory and white.

Warm Spring Characteristics

Skin Tone: Creamy white, ivory, and peach with golden undertones

Eye Color: Hazel, blue green, blue, turquoise or golden brown

Hair Color: Blond, flaxen, strawberry red, golden gray, golden brown

Suggested Fashion Colors: Warm hues like camel, peach, ivory, apricot, yellows, golden browns, apple green, leaf green and spring blues. *Avoid dark dull hues and shades.*

Warm Autumn Characteristics

Skin Tone: Beige, gold, copper with golden undertones

Eye Color: Hazel, amber, golden to dark brown, green, turquoise

Hair Color: Auburn, red chestnut, ginger, golden-brown, gray and brunettes

Suggested Fashion Colors: Earthy and spicy colors like camel, golden warm and dark browns, orange, rust and red, kelly, forest, avocado and moss greens. *Avoid blue tones such as navy.*

Cool Summer Characteristics

Skin Color: Pale or rosy beige, light olive with blue or pink undertones

Eye Color: Blue, gray blue, gray, green, and hazel

Hair Color: Natural blonds, light brown, dark brown, brunette, gray, blue gray

Suggested Fashion Colors: Pastels and soft neutrals with blue and pink undertones like rose, pink and dusty pinks, mauve, burgundy, soft blues, soft greens, lavender, plum, rose-brown, taupe and grays. *Black could be harsh.*

Cool Winter Characteristics

Skin Tone: Porcelain, golden olive, dark olive, brown, dark brown and black

Eye Color: Dark brown, dark blue, violet

Hair Color: Black, blue black, ash, brown and silver

Suggested Fashion Colors: Sharp and clear colors like red, shocking pink, royal blue, sapphire, dark blue, navy blue, teal, green, and black, whites and icy lighter tints. *Pastels don't work as well.*

Monochromatic

A way to feel chic and elegant while looking slimmer and taller at the same time is to dress monochromatically—wearing one color from head to toe creates a strong unbroken vertical line that gives the illusion of added inches. Try this amazingly simple yet stylish way of dressing in one of your core colors. Monochromatic dressing will extend your wardrobe and make your life less complicated; but, like anything, don't overdo it. If this becomes a signature for your style try different fabric textures and patterns in the same color to add dimension and dramatic sophistication. If you've never tried dressing monochromatically you will find it to be very natural, so take advantage of it. ***Try this**: If you're a "spring" try dressing in all camel or golden brown; if you're an "autumn" try dressing in all rust or golden brown; if you're a "summer" try dressing in all dusty pinks and grays; and if you're a "winter" try dressing in all icy pink, red or black.*

A Color's Personality

White: represents light, goodness, innocence, purity, virginity, perfection, safety, cleanliness and faith.

Pink: represents femininity, love, romance, friendship and passiveness.

Yellow: represents sunshine, joy, happiness freshness and energy.

Green: represents nature, harmony, freshness, safety, fertility, growth and money.

Dark Green: represents, money, ambition, greed, and jealousy.

Olive Green: represents peace and commitment.

Gold: represents illumination, wisdom, prestige and high quality.

Orange: represents energy, happiness, joy, sunshine and the tropics.

Red Orange: represents energy, sexual passion, pleasure, desire and aggression.

Red: represents energy, intensity, power, determination, passion, desire and love.

Light Red: represents sensitivity, passion, joy and love.

Dark Red: represents, willpower, leadership, courage, vigor and rage.

Reddish Brown: represents harvest and fall.

Brown: represents stability.

Blue: represents the sky, the sea, trust, loyalty, confidence, intelligence, faith, truth and heaven.

Light Blue: represents tranquility, peace, softness, healing and health.

Dark Blue: represents power, integrity knowledge, seriousness and trustworthiness.

Aqua: represents harmony, emotional healing and protection.

Purple: represents energy, stability, creativity, royalty, power, wisdom and dignity.

Light Purple: represents romance and love.

Dark Purple: represents sadness and gloom.

Black: represents elegance, power, prestige, formality, strength, authority, mystery and death.

Fashion is a versatile yet complex language

For Every Occasion

For every occasion there is a proper way to dress. Understanding the rules from the list below will help you to see where you may want to start working to build your authentic wardrobe.

Evening Attire

White Tie is as beautiful and fabulous as formal can be. An ultra feminine full-length evening dress is a must. Your counterpart would wear a tailcoat. No options. Who knows, maybe you are aspiring to work with the United Nations where you'll be invited to white tie events with dignitaries and royalties, raising money and awareness for your special causes.

Black Tie is formal and gowns are still the protocol; however, being as relaxed as we are today, a beautiful evening pantsuit or spectacular skirt and blouse would be lovely as well. Your counterpart would wear a tuxedo.

Semi-Formal/Cocktail is a relaxed but elegant look. A short dress is appropriate, which could be in a variety of shapes and lengths. The "little black dress" is a favorite. Your counterpart would wear an evening jacket.

Dressy Casual is a casual but elegant look. Semi-dressy fabrics are used in pantsuits, dresses and coordinated separates. Well-coordinated shoes and accessories are a must.

Business Attire

Power Business/The Executive Look is usually a feminine skirt suit or tailored dress of quality fabrics and excellent workmanship. Beautiful and elegant, yet conservative accessories are a must. Feminine does not mean seductive.

General Business is the middle ground of office and business attire. Individual pieces can work together to suit up in without feeling suited up. A relaxed yet tailored pantsuit or less-constructed skirt suit works well.

Business Casual is dressing professionally and feeling more relaxed in your clothes, while at the same time maintaining personal power by being neat and pulled together. You may select a dress, a pantsuit, a skirt and blouse ensemble or slacks and twin set. Be creative—the key is looking good while feeling relaxed and professional.

Casual Chic is taking a fabulous piece, like a beautiful silk top and mixing it with jeans and a fabulous pair of shoes. When you think of casual chic, think easy separates, textured pieces and contrasting fabrics: leathers, velvets, silks, lace, sparkly tops and sateen pants. All are great pieces to include in your wardrobe if you work in creative industries or less traditional fields.

Sports and Play Attire

Active Casual allows you to get your cardiovascular health up to speed and look good while you're doing it. These are clothes worn for active sports, working out and playing—jogging suits, sweat suits, tennis skirts, work-out clothes, running shorts and leggings are all appropriate in the gym or at the coffee shop and running quick errands.

Sporty Casual is not about you playing a sport it's about you choosing the look of a spectator, just hanging out or running extended errands. This look includes jeans, cotton pants, shorts, a button-down, tees and polo-style shirts to name a few—and don't forget the appropriate casual shoes.

Sporty Chic is cool and simple. You look like you're headed to or leaving the country club all the time but you never sweat. The tops are light-colored and fitted, polo style. Skirts are short and pants are cropped. The shoes are light-weight stylish sneakers or simple, well-made leather thongs, always showing that perfect pedicure. Accessories include oversized sunglasses, canvas totes and any discreet hi-tech gadget.

Urban Casual is trendy, casual street glamour for the younger crowd. It's mixing designer high-fashion pieces with athletic and sports wear. It's hip hop starlets setting street trends that soon find themselves in night clubs and stores across America.

Intimate Apparel

I love it when I'm relaxing, alone at home, or on vacation with my husband and children when I get to lie around in the most exquisite silks and cottons for days, rejuvenating my whole self by totally relaxing. These are the times that I believe intimate apparel is immensely important and a must-have.

Lounge Wear was designed to recline and lie around in for comfort, such as flowing house gowns, robes, housecoats, muumuus, bed jackets, dusters, nursing gowns and pool attire.

Lingerie is women's undergarments, such as panties, bras, slips, camisoles, girdles, pajamas and night gowns. These garments are to be worn underneath your outerwear and in your bedroom. However, today, the lines between lingerie and ready-to-wear apparel are blurred. Designers are creating cross-over looks that can double as cocktail dresses. But, darling, please use your best judgment before stepping outside of your *chamber à coucher* in your lingerie.

Body Types and Shapes Revisited

Now that we've gone through *occasions* and the appropriate attire for certain events, and *clothing personality types*, the style of clothing that best suits your ideal self and helps you to express yourself authentically, I want to revisit the basics of *body types and shapes*. This, in my opinion is the catalyst in you being able to create and perfect your authentic image with style, confidence and ease. These components will be followed by *lifestyles*—the way you're living. The goal is to help you to develop a clear picture of how these elements come together to play an integral part in you *getting ready and perfecting your authentic image…* daily. If you need more information on body types and body shapes refer to Chapter 2.

***Remember** the body types**
The **ectomorphic** body type is usually tall and thin with long legs and a relatively flat chest.

The **mesomorphic** body type is usually athletic, hard and muscular with broad shoulders and a medium to large chest.

The **endomorphic** body type is usually heavily boned and rounded in appearance, especially around the abdominal area with fuller bosoms.
**most of us are combinations of the above, with one being more dominate.*

The **Pear** shape has a slim upper body, a small waist and voluptuous hips and thighs. Your neck may be one of your best assets.

The **Inverted Pear** shape has a larger upper body characterized by fuller shoulders, larger bust and a narrow lower body. Your bottom and legs have the potential to look fabulous forever.

The **Apple** shape is top-heavy with a fuller mid-section and breasts that are wider than your hips. You have a flat bottom with nice, relatively thin thighs and legs that could serve you well.

The **Slender** shape is fairly equal in the chest, waist and hips. You are straight up and down, like a ruler for the most part.

The **Hourglass** shape has balanced shoulders and hips, with a small waist. Your silhouette is harmonious, curvaceous and feminine.

The **Balanced** shape is the same size on top and bottom. The slender balanced shaped woman is the easiest to dress. Most high-fashion designers create designs with this body shape in mind.

The dress must not hang on the body but follow its lines.
—Madeleine Vionnet

Clothing Lines

"Silhouette" has always been one of my favorite fashion words to say out loud. There is something romantic and elegant about the way it forms in my mouth and glides out as if I were about to sing a love song. Also, I like the thought of my silhouette being outlined, in life size, giving me a fabulous view of every visual line and curve of my body. That's what designers do when they design. They consider *style lines, design lines and detail lines* to establish the shape and mood of each piece designed.

Visual Lines

Style Lines are formed by the outlines of garments. They can enhance, alter or conceal your silhouette. For instance, a high-waisted Empire style can camouflage a thick or wide waistline. An A-Line style can hide broad or wide hips and the blouson style gives the appearance of fuller breasts.

Design Lines are strong lines created within the style of the garment. They can add curves, height, length and width to your silhouette. Fabulous illusions have been created using layers, pleats, openings, pockets, prints and accessories… artfully created using design lines.

Detail Lines are lines that affect lengths, hemlines, sleeves, fabrics and textures of the garment.

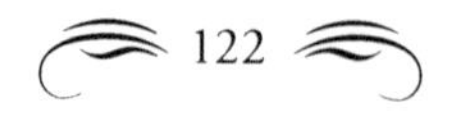

Design Lines Can Include:

- *Vertical Lines* give the illusion of height and slenderness—elongating.
- *Diagonal Lines* have two illusions—a short diagonal line is more horizontal, creating the illusion of width. A longer diagonal line is more vertical in its illusion, adding length.
- *Horizontal Lines* broaden and shorten, adding the illusion of width.
- *Curved Lines* can redefine your silhouette by emphasizing roundness and softness.

When it comes to building your wardrobe and looking your very best, understanding your body's lines (your silhouette or body shape and proportions) and how they correlate with the lines of clothing is one of the most important aspects of *getting ready*. Using these lines effectively can help you create flattering illusions that will distract from your physical flaws while enhancing your personal assets.

When I am in the mood to look impressively feminine and elegant, my first consideration is a silk, satin or jersey dress that is cut on the bias. I know this style will accentuate my silhouette, allowing the fabric to cling softly while draping fluidly across my body for maximum slink appeal. For this reason I love the bias cut and I am in complete agreement with Madeleine Vionnet, the French designer who revolutionized this way of cutting and designing, when she said, "The dress must not hang on the body but follow its lines. It must accompany its wearer and when a woman smiles the dress must smile with her." That means you're wearing the dress, darling—the dress is not wearing you.

Part Three

The unexamined wardrobe is not worth wearing.

Chapter 8
Out of the Closet

My closet, like many of my clients' closets, is a well-guarded intimate space that is full of secretive feminine power. It is a space where I feel free to pray and have conversations with God, to reflect and to visualize. It is a space where I conjure up my wildest girlish and romantic fantasies. When I go into my closet, I can be *me*. My husband and children are not welcomed there. It's cozy and sacred and I hide all sorts of tangible and intangible things there. I have had large *boudoirs* that included chaise lounges, exquisite art and chilled beverages. I have also had closets that were so small I could barely squeeze inside. What I know for sure is that every closet, regardless of its size, can be neat, functional and inviting. It can contain space enough to hang and store a fabulous basic wardrobe, allowing you to step out with style whenever you choose.

Like many of my clients, I sometimes find myself holding onto things in my closet and my drawers a little too long. Not the photographs or the chocolates—but clothes that I'm not going to wear anymore or clothes that should never have landed in my closet in the first place. So, at least once a year I force myself to evaluate and audit my own closet. I encourage you to do this as well. This process also includes getting rid of old lingerie, lounge wear, hose and socks.

Women usually love what they buy, yet hate two-thirds of what is in their closets.
—Mignon McLaughlin

The Audit

In giving yourself permission to complete a thorough closet evaluation and audit, you must be bold and honest with yourself about certain clothes and items in your closet. Otherwise you'll run the risk of not making much progress.

I want you to:

- Take away all of the clothing and accessories that you really dislike.
- Take away the pieces that you realized were mistakes the moment you left the store.
- Take away the gifts that you have never worn or used.
- Take away all other garments that you know you'll never wear again.
- Take away all of the clothes that are incongruent with your authentic fashion personality.
- Take away all of the clothes that you absolutely adore but you know you will never fit into again.
- Take away all of the clothes that have unflattering lines, patterns and colors.
- Take out all of the clothes that are really outdated.
- Take out all of your stained, torn or irreparable clothing.

- **G**et rid of all abused, old and run over shoes.
- **G**et rid of all old and damaged handbags and belts.
- **T**ake out all of your old coats.
- **A**udit and organize your jewelry.
- **T**ake away all the unnecessary junk—wire hangers, empty shoe and hat boxes, shopping bags, plastic, etc.

It is amazing what a good tailor can do to make an old jacket look new again.

Lifestyle Grouping

To Do List:

- **S**eparate what's left of your wardrobe into a pile for each area of your life: work, sports, evening, lounging, gardening, etc. (this will depend on your lifestyle. Some pieces will probably overlap).
- **T**ry on every piece for proper fit. Then ask yourself, "Why did I keep this piece? Does it feel good on? Does it make me feel good? Does it look fabulous on me? If you still love it, keep it. If it needs tweaking, have it altered. If you don't like it, donate it.
- **M**odernize your older, fabulous pieces by tweaking through alterations:
  - **A**djusting the hem
  - **R**emoving the collar
  - **C**hanging the shape
  - **C**hanging the belt
  - **R**emoving or adding shoulder pads
  - **C**hanging the buttons—you get the picture.
- **L**ist and record everything that you have in each category. This includes clothing, shoes, coats, lingerie and accessories.
- **M**easure how you stack up in each category. This list will give you your foundation—your core wardrobe.
- **N**ow you're ready to create new outfits from clothes that you already have and really like.

Stepping into your closet right after your audit might seem a little scary at first, but don't be discouraged. Even if you're on a tight budget, you'll be able to build a fabulously stylish wardrobe designed around it, your body shape, your fashion personality type and your lifestyle in about two to three short seasons. *If you plan on looking consistently great then it's a good idea to build a special relationship with a tailor for A-1 alterations and a proper dry cleaner to take care of your special fashion needs.*

Ready to Shop

Now, when you are ready to incorporate new, exciting pieces into your existing wardrobe you'll have a well-thought-out plan. Instead of feeling like an impossible chore, your shopping experience can be exhilarating and rewarding—you'll know exactly what you're looking for, and you'll save money and spend less time by *not* going to stores that *don't* have the type of clothing that fits into your fashion personality type.

- **R**efer to the list you made during your closet audit.
- **G**o through the list again and decide what it is that you'd like to buy to complete or add to your wardrobe.
- **S**et your budget.

You don't need more money or more time to look consistently great—you need style!

Getting Ready Chloé-Style starts long before you step into your closet to begin the process of putting together your core wardrobe—it starts the moment you commit to being an IBBer. Getting Ready Chloé-Style starts with you feeling good about who you are as a woman and who you're being in the world. It starts with self-love, with you appreciating your body and all your positive attributes. The getting dressed of *getting ready* is the last step of the process, the icing on the cake, so to speak. Something that flows harmonious with your personality and your lifestyle shouldn't take too much thought on a daily basis—but you look like you do because you always manage to present yourself in a poised, polished and put-together way.

Your goal: *To walk into your closet at any given time, for any occasion that goes along with your authentic lifestyle and walk out looking like a million bucks—from the most casual to the most elegant.*

Complete the exercise below to acquire a sense of style and build a fabulous wardrobe for that just right look... every time.

1. What is your fashion personality type?

____

2. What is your body type?

____

3. What is your shape?

____

4. What are your proportions?

Height_____________

Weight_____________

Frame size__________

5. What are your best core colors: black, brown, blue, navy, gray, taupe, camel, ivory or white?

a. Select two or three (core) dark colors and a (core) light color that coordinate, based on your *"season." For example, I am a cool "winter," so I would choose my favorite colors—a fabulous shade of red, black and ivory—great workable colors for me. Of course, I would incorporate other colors as my budget permits me to develop my new wardrobe.*

____

____

____

____

____

b. Select your accent colors (bold, pastels, icy, etc).

____

____

____

6. Maximize your resources by playing up your strengths and positive traits. What are they?

____

____

____

____

____

____

____

a. Camouflage any negative or unfavorable traits. What are they?

____

____

____

7. Your wardrobe foundation should consist of quality classic pieces of related colors that harmonize, coordinate or accent.

a. Don't be afraid to use different textures and patterns and a mixture of fabrics to add style.

b. Choose your jackets, skirts, and pants in your dark or neutral colors.

c. Choose your blouses, tops, shirts and sweaters in your accent colors.

d. Again, always buy the best quality you can afford. In fashion and style, quality is always better than quantity.

8. Shop based on your lifestyle.

a. How do you spend most of your time?

b. What will you wear most often?

c. Invest wisely—will you wear a pair of quality basic pumps more often than a fabulous high-tea hat?

Lifestyle Examples

Isabella, an attorney, spends most days in meetings and professional settings. Her core wardrobe consists of executive business attire which spills over into her social evening. Isabella knows that dressing monochromatically works for her apple shape, giving her one continuous flow of color, helping her to appear taller and leaner. She also knows to avoid high-waisted skirts and pants that make her waist look even shorter.

Hannah, a special education teacher with a horse farm, has a core wardrobe that consists of sporty casual attire and a few dressy casual pieces for weekends. Hannah knows that V-necks and wrap dresses are wonderful and easy for her hourglass body shape. She also knows to stay away from anything that does not accentuate her waist. *You'll learn more about these two women and others later.*

10. Stick with the lines, cuts and styles that work for you.

11. Follow trends without being trendy—then incorporate your style of the trend into your wardrobe and step out looking fabulous and *so you,* every day.

Fashion and Style Basics

1. Appropriate undergarments are a must—the goal is to maintain a smooth, uplifted and enhanced foundation.

2. A classic three-piece black suit in lightweight wool or silk. The look that works best for most is a cinched-waist jacket, an A-line or pencil skirt and flared slacks; even if you're far from traditional business this staple will definitely come in handy and will extend your wardrobe.

3. A cool cinched-waist jacket in a fabulous color and fabric.

4. A pair of black or dark-wash boot-cut jeans.

5. A medium or light-colored tailored A-line or pencil skirt in lightweight wool or silk (coordinates with cinched-waist jacket).

6. An evening skirt in black (leather, tiered, asymmetrical. pleated, floral, lace, etc, depending on your fashion personality type).

7. A classic white shirt—with or without cuffs.

8. A rich creamy silk camisole.

9. A black lace shell.

10. A black or cream mock neck fitted silk sweater.

11. A striped tee.

12. A geometric or floral fitted silk blouse (coordinates with cinched waist jacket and black suit).

13. A classic twin set in a beautiful jewel tone, icy or pastel.

14. A fabulous little black dress.

15. A fabulous black handbag for day time.

16. A fabulous little evening bag.

17. A quality black leather belt.

18. A pair of fabulous, yet comfortable black leather pumps or sling-backs.

19. A pair of chic black flats.

20. Your signature jewelry—depending on your fashion personality type: pearls add elegance, while chunky bangles add character to a bohemian look.

21. A glowing complexion and beautiful make-up.

22. A fabulous hairstyle.

23. Neat hands and nails.

24. A winning personality and attitude.

25. A determined ideal, set goals and a strategic plan to get you there once you're dressed and ready to go! *Substitute colors based on your best workable core colors.*

With these fashion and style basics, you will have a great foundation for the start of a versatile wardrobe. Remember, when establishing or updating your wardrobe, it is a good idea to look at mannequins in stores and fashion magazines to see how colors and fabrics are coordinated and to get ideas for styling. However, keep in mind that what works well in photographs may not work well in real life.

Use your friends to help you see how you can arrange and coordinate your existing pieces in ways that you may not have thought of and to gain a fresh outlook. You don't have to rush out to buy everything all at once. Incorporate a few pieces at a time into your existing wardrobe to expand your closet. Keep in mind that simply updating your accessories can be a cost-effective way to follow the latest trends and styles.

Along with wardrobe, paying close attention to grooming, body shape, size and fashion adornment will generate more positive behavior. A satisfied self exudes increased self-esteem. When we care about ourselves, others can sense it and they'll treat us with more respect.

How to Find Your Signature Fashion and Style Basics

Boutiques

When you find a little shop that caters to your fashion personality type you'd better be careful. It can be intoxicating, and even addictive. The most fabulous and amazing are calling themselves lifestyle boutiques. Your favorite little shops will have that *it* piece for you almost every time you stop by. The most personal boutiques buy particular items from show rooms with *you* in mind, inform you of sales, and, if you're a favorite, they'll even send loads of amazing pieces and outfits to your home for fittings... unless, of course, you're the type who enjoys being seen at the coolest fashion spots in town. In most cases the merchandise at boutiques is not one-of-a-kind. However, they are unique and quite special.

Catalogs

Many of your favorite specialty stores and boutiques have fabulous catalogs today and I'll be the first to admit it. I love flipping through the slick pages. They can be enticing. After receiving a catalog from a local boutique recently, I was so impressed I stopped by the store the very next day for a unique *must-have* that I needed to include in my wardrobe, only to find a few other fashionable women clamoring for the same item. They had received the catalog, too. Today, catalog shoppers are savvy shoppers, finding stylish, unique merchandise.

Consignment Shops

A wonderful way to look fabulous all the time without breaking your bank account is shopping consignment and resale stores. Like any store or boutique, you'll want to know which shops suit your taste and fashion personality type. The best consignment shops provide personal service that you'll love. By getting on the mailing list and getting to know the sales staff, you'll be one of the first to hear about promotions and sales. Otherwise you'll need to stop in often to find the best merchandise. Try everything on and look in different sizes. Some items have been altered and you probably won't be able to return them. Don't forget to look for accessories while you're there. You'll pay a fraction of the original price for the same quality and style.

Custom Designers

Some of the most exciting fashion experiences I've had involved having clothes designed and fitted especially for my body. As a model in Milan, one of my favorite designers to work for was Gian Franco Ferré. The fittings were as exciting as the Prêt-à-Porter show itself. The experience of having two to five outfits designed and fitted with my body in mind was extraordinary, especially when Signior Ferré would ask, "Chloé, what do you think? How do you feel in the outfit?" Custom designs can be for any fashion personality type, allowing you to have input to how you want your wardrobe or special outfits to look, flow and feel. It can be pricy but is absolutely based on your fashion personality type, your body type, shape and lifestyle. I recommend the experience for everyone—at least once.

Department Stores

Everything from cosmetics to dishwashers has been purchased at department stores. If you're the type who loves one-stop shopping, if you know what you want and have no need to spend a lot of time browsing, then department store shopping may suit you well. To make it count though, it's a good idea to know the department store's audience before heading out to one. You'll want to make sure it suits your taste and budget. Sears and J.C. Penny cater to a particular audience. Bloomingdale's, Nordstrom, Macy's, Neiman Marcus and Bergdorf Goodman cater to a certain audience as well and can be referred to as *Specialty Stores.* They don't offer appliances and other home wares but they do offer special services like trunk shows and personal appearances from designers, quaint cafes, entertainment, salespeople that go out of their way for you and personal shoppers.

Discount Stores

Who doesn't love a good deal, especially when it comes to fashion? Today, more of us are looking for offers we can't refuse and discounters from Target, T.J. Maxx, Loehmann's and Filene's Basement, to name a few, are all competing to satisfy our desires. If you have the time it takes to browse and a good eye, you can unearth wonderful designer deals at discount stores. But, plan to visit often and make friends with one of the salespersons to get the inside scoop on new shipments.

Malls

Today's malls are sophisticated gathering spaces filled with friends hooking up for coffee at Starbucks and families shopping, eating and taking in a movie, or two. Professional divas can have their spa and salon needs taken care of in the morning, conduct a power lunch meeting at the new "in" restaurant at noon, then head over to the Armani boutique to pick up a new suit that has been altered to fit her body. Like your favorite department store, your favorite mall will depend upon where you live and your lifestyle, as well as your fashion personality type and budget. With everything under one roof, going to the mall can be a bona fide social happening. I love watching the people. Expect to pay more.

Outlet Shopping

If you want substantial savings, good-quality merchandise and an extensive selection, then outlet shopping might be your thing—if you don't mind last season's merchandise and you're not looking to be voted the trendiest person in town. These savings can be passed on to us for several reasons. First, there are outlet-only lines that are slightly different from regular store lines—maybe a lesser-quality fabric or lower quality buttons are used. Secondly, there is no middleman involved. Outlet merchandise is shipped right from the factories to the outlets and some of the merchandise might be slightly flawed. For these reasons you can save up to thirty to fifty percent on fabulous fashions. Like the malls, outlet shopping can be an event in and of itself, especially when you factor in the drive it usually takes to get there.

Vintage Stores

If you're a trendsetter who loves one-of-a-kind pieces from another era, and you hate the thought of showing up looking predictable or, even worse, being dressed like someone else, then you might like vintage shopping. Real vintage can come from designers' high fashion collections, women's custom designs, good-quality brand names and good-quality no names. The thread that runs through all vintage is high quality and desirability.

Web Shopping

Today, because of the internet there are sky malls—virtual shopping spaces where you have options to browse hundreds of stores and view thousands of products, right from the privacy of your own home or office or wherever you can take a wireless computer or handheld device. Literally, a world of options awaits you with a click of your mouse. If you're the type who gets a certain high in seeing the UPS guy at your front door, then this type of shopping can feed into your addiction, so be careful. On the other hand, if you're the type who has very little time for shopping, then this new way of shopping can work beautifully with your lifestyle. Also, I've seen virtual shopping work well for clients who may have a few body image issues and want to try clothes on at home. I have learned from my teenage son as well, who seems to be able to find anything that he wants to buy from e-Bay and East Bay, and usually for a fraction of the cost. Everything can be found and purchased through Web shopping, from food to furniture and everything in between.

Shopping Tips

- •Think of your overall direction and fashion personality type.
- •Stick to your budget.
- •Stick to your plan and only buy what's on your list.
- •Wear comfortable, but stylish clothes that are easy to take off and put on.
- •Don't wait until the last minute to shop for what you really need.
- •Don't be misled by a sale—unless, of course, it has exactly what's on your list.
- •Look for quality over quantity.
- •Try everything on and look in a full-length three-way mirror.
- •Test for comfort and functionality by sitting and bending.
- •Ask yourself—can the garment breathe, can I exhale in this?
- •Does the garment or outfit need alterations?
- •Make friends with special salespersons at your favorite stores and ask them to contact you when items you would like go on sale or when the store has new arrivals.
- •Ask if you can return items.
- •Does it look absolutely fabulous on you?
- •And finally, does it fit into your plan of how you'd like others to perceive you based on your goals?

Make sure you have the appropriate undergarments on your shopping list and, if you've never been measured properly for your bra size, get fitted.

Buying the Right Undergarments

A **bra** or **brassiere** is a lingerie item that can accentuate, lift and support the bust and take the strain off the connective tissue. It

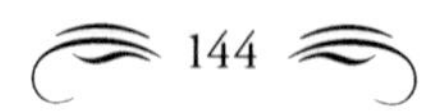

can be closed in the front or in the back; the straps can be central, lateral, crossed or strapless. There are a variety of bra designs that can fit everyone's need and bodice design—*just make sure your bra fits properly.*

Types of Bras

1. **Adhesive Bra**: A strapless, backless self-adhesive silicone bra designed to wear under backless and strapless clothing.
2. **Athletic Bra:** A bra that provides additional support for breast tissue worn during active sports and working out.
3. **Bustier:** A strapless bra that stretches to the waist and may have garters at the bottom.
4. **Convertible Bra:** A bra designed with straps that can be moved, removed, and/or adjusted to accommodate a halter, strapless, crisscross or open back.
5. **Demi-Cup Bra:** A bra that gives breasts a boost and reveals the upper portion of the breast—perfect for wearing under low-cut dresses and button-downs.
6. **Enhancing Bra:** A bra that makes the breast look bigger by pulling up and in, and padding from below. Wonderful for small-breasted women.
7. **Front Closure Bra:** A bra that snaps or hooks in the front. Fabulous for plunging necklines.
8. **Minimizer Bra:** A bra that reduces the appearance of a large-breasted woman, making the breast seem smaller by using sturdy fabric and wide back and shoulder straps.
9. **Molded-Cup Bra:** A smooth opaque bra that supports and defines. Wonderful under Tee-shirts and smooth tops.

10. **Push-Up Bra:** A bra designed to support and lift, increasing the appearance of the bust size and revealing more cleavage through padding. The bust can be partly or fully covered.
11. **Racerback Bra:** A bra that supports and crosses in the back, Good for sports and racerback tanks.
12. **Seamless Bra:** A smooth, comfortable bra without seams.
13. **Shelf Bra:** A bra that rests under the breast to push up and support without covering the nipples.
14. **Silicone-Cup Bra:** A bra with cups that contain silicone padding.
15. **Strapless Bra:** A bra with wide sides to keep the bra in place. It can have detachable straps that can be modified into a halter-style bra. Wonderful with spaghetti traps and party dresses.
16. **Underwire Bra:** A bra with thin wire sewn into the lower portion of the cups for additional support. Fabulous for larger-breasted women.

Panties are a woman's essential item and seem to be in every lady's lingerie drawer. They can be seamless, sheer, full, long leg, high rise and even barely there.

Types of Panties

1. **Boy Briefs:** Similar to hip briefs but tend to have more leg in them while hip briefs are cut higher; work well under light summer skirts and dresses.
2. **Bikini:** Bikinis have a full seat, are cut at the thigh and are generally mid-to low-rise.

3. **High-Rise Briefs:** Underwear that comes up to the belly button or higher, they have a full and roomy seat and hit the thigh. They are the most conservative of all underwear.
4. **Low-Rise Hip Briefs:** Provide a full seat and coverage and a cool laid-back sporty look, cut more like shorts, they are comfortable and fun—great to wear under jeans and for working out.
5. **String Bikini:** a bikini with an elastic string that allows for added comfort.
6. **Tanga:** A lingerie pant style that has thin straps across the hips, similar to boy briefs but slightly higher in the waist and lower in the leg, with nearly a full seat.
7. **Tap Pants:** A lingerie pant style with loose-fitting legs and a slightly smaller seat which usually goes higher on the sides.
8. **Thin Seamless Briefs:** Provide a full seat and coverage and works well with silky skirts and thin pants.
9. **Thongs:** Usually worn to prevent visible panty lines.
    a. **Rio Thong:** This is the most popular style of thong, with straps that rise up on the sides.
    b. **T-Back Thong:** A thong that forms a perfect "T" shape in the back.
    c. **G-String Thong:** Is strictly string, with no coverage at all. The least comfortable.

Other Undergarments

1. **Stretchy Camisole:** Lingerie that is worn under sheer tops.
2. **Silk Camisole:** A short loose-fitting lingerie top that ends at the waistline: can be worn under outer garments to protect skin or worn visibly under an open jacket.

3. **Half Slip:** Silky lingerie that looks like a full skirt: keeps clingy skirts from sticking to your legs.
4. **Waist Shaper:** Lingerie that shapes and controls the waist.
5. **Tummy-Control Briefs:** High-rise brief panties that smooth and control the tummy.
6. **Leg Shapers:** Light-weight, sturdy Capri-type control panties.

Perfecting Your Authentic Image

In order to fully and effectively demonstrate the process of creating and perfecting your authentic image, I have strategically designed six images of women. *The personification and story for each of them are composites; individual names and identifying characteristics have been invented by me for the sole purpose of illustration—to show you what it takes for an image enhancement specialist to attain high levels of success in assisting each client to create and perfect her authentic image. Nevertheless, these personifications reflect the authentic situations, careers and lifestyles of hundreds of women. If you think you recognize yourself in the pages, the similarities are strictly coincidental. However, my goal is that one of these incredible women just might empower and/or inspire you.*

Madison, Ava, Isabella, Angela, Hannah and Rebecca are my *Getting Ready Girls*—and through each of them I will demonstrate the process of how to create a basic wardrobe that can be transformed into dozens of outfit combinations that take each of them where they want to go—all while presenting a trustworthy appearance. Each image will be enhanced based on individual body type and shape, height, size, age, career and lifestyle. My hope is that you can find a little bit of yourself in one of them, or perhaps in traits from two or more of them to help you develop your personal style and create dozens of outfits and outfit combinations that are just right for you.

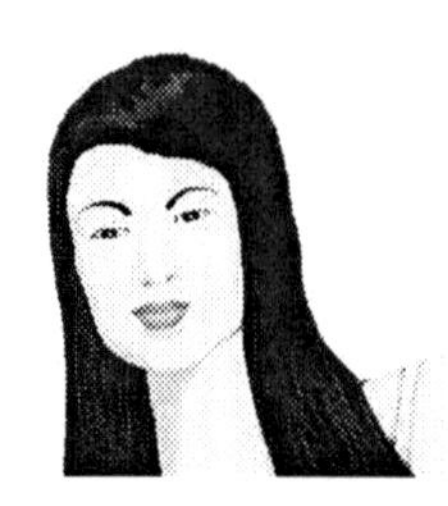

Madison is a twenty-two-year-old eccentric lover of everything art, including traveling to exotic places collecting exquisite paintings, drawings, sculptures and other fine art. She has worked as an art dealer since age nineteen, closing five-figure art deals for her grandparents' art gallery and business. Madison lives in a midtown loft near her family's business. She is confident, strong, beautiful, focused and opinionated—she does not want her age, slender body and girlish looks to get in the way of being taken seriously in the competitive world of art. Her challenge is to look more poised and professional while negotiating amazing art deals. On the other hand, she wants to maintain her authenticity and self-expression.

Madison is fun to be around and always receives more than enough invitations to have a fabulous meal with family and friends. She does not cook but keeps plenty of fresh fruits and healthy snacks in her minimalist loft. She drinks plenty of water and fresh-squeezed juice daily. Speed walking and running around the park with Mister, her American Eskimo Spitz, energizes her.

Going to art exhibits and gallery openings is part of Madison's work and she loves every minute of it. Photography is what she shines in personally and she loves sharing it with middle-school children through an after-school program she created and funds. Madison is admired by many—the children she empowers, her parents and friends, and professionals in the art world. My job is to create a professional look for Madison... one that gives curves to her slender body type, incorporates her Bohemian fashion personality, maintains her youth and adds a level of professionalism as a representative of her grandparents' art business. *Check out Madison's personification and review the necessary information it takes to design, create and perfect an empowering image which still maintains her authenticity.*

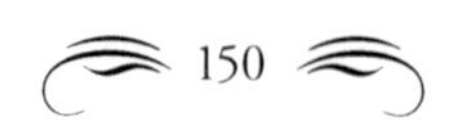

Madison's Personification

Age Height Weight

22 5'2" 108

Size Frame

2/4 Small

Body Type Body Shape

Ectomorphic Slender

Challenge

Looks sixteen—not polished

Career Choice

Art Dealer

Lifestyle

Madison is an energetic, healthy and fit, single, urban, minimalist who loves laughing, quality living and international experiences.

Fashion Personality Type

Bohemian and Casual

Color Season

Cool winter—porcelain skin, dark brown eyes and black hair.

Madison in Business Casual Attire

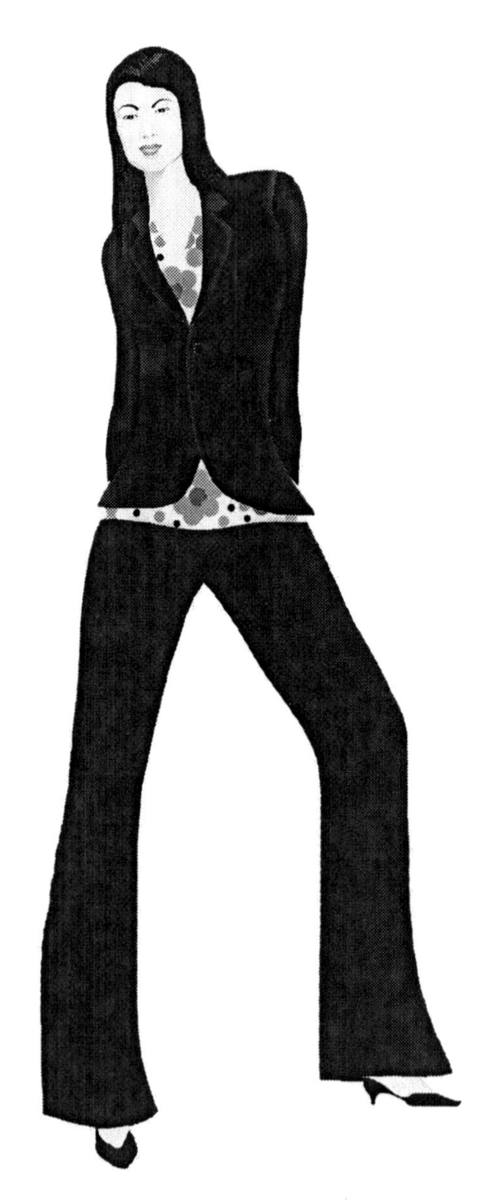

Madison's self expression in fashion is bohemian and relaxed. Because of her slender, petite body, she often makes the mistake of wearing oversized jackets and tops with long flowing skirts—which makes her petite body appear even shorter and disheveled. I will create the illusion of extra inches and curves for her while allowing her fashion personality to peak through as she projects a professional authentic image—one that is acceptable in dealing with the more mature individuals of the high-end art business.

1.First and foremost, Madison must wear clothes that fit her petite body.

2.She loves black, so I've selected a black pants suit for her in high-quality, seasonally versatile worsted wool.

3.The shoulders of the jacket define Madison's shoulders.

4. The slightly cinched waist gives the illusion of a waist line.
5. The jacket length elongates her short torso.
6. The flared, cuffless pants make her legs look longer.
7. The black higher-heeled shoes make her look taller.
8. The V-neck patterned halter pulls the eye down vertically and adds just enough color and a touch of bohemian flair.

This polished easygoing work look will serve Madison well and help her to close many more five-figure art deals.

Madison's Fashion and Style Checklist:

1. Black classic structured suit with boot cut pants in light-weight wool
2. Yellow bomber jacket
3. Yellow and orange silk floral halter top
4. White eyelet cinched waist tank
5. White bell-sleeved tunic in cotton and lace
6. White cotton wrap blouse—elbow length
7. Black-and-white, wide horizontal striped boatneck tee
8. Black, shocking pink and white long-sleeved graphic print silk blouse
9. Black long-sleeved turtle neck sweater
10. Black, yellow and orange floral print halter shift dress
11. Dark wash, mid-rise, skinny jeans
12. Black knee-length, A-line vintage-y skirt with yellow floral print
13. Red cotton tiered skirt
14. Black mid-heel boots
15. Black low-heel d'orsay
16. Silver flat strappy sandals
17. Silver bangles and silver hoop earrings
18. Black ethnic belt
19. Black fringed oversized hippie bag with shoulder straps
20. Enhancing bras

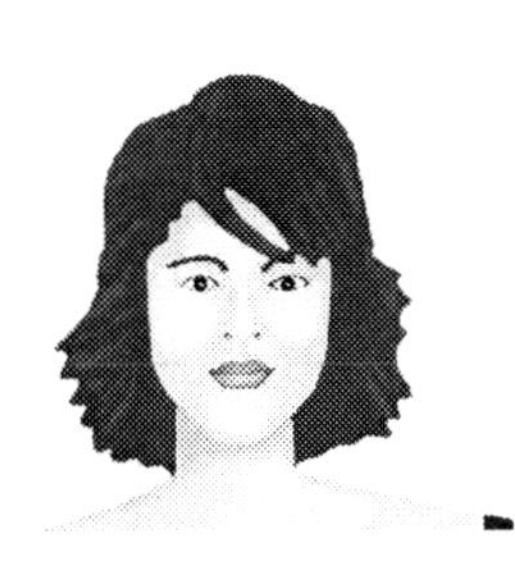

Ava has a sincere and intense passion for classic black-and-white films and art deco, jewelry, furniture and antiques. This infatuation was passed down from her fabulous and beloved great-grandmother, Stella. Ava's life-long fascination with the movies, fashions and art that her great-grandmother adored spilled over into her life goals, sending her to Florence to study cinematography and film production to become a sought-after film and video editor. At twenty-eight years old, Ava has acquired a bold, take-charge personality. She is determined, driven and focused. After seven years of working for a major production company, she now provides independent editing services for directors for movies and videos through her home studio. Ava is as glamorous as the starlets in the old black-and-white films she loves. Her image challenge is to consistently camouflage a short waist and to perfect a *dressed down* yet glamorous look that works with her lifestyle. Ava's long, elegant and shapely legs are tremendous assets.

Ava and Paolo, her husband of two years, share a Mediterranean lifestyle. They live in town in an airy Craftsman bungalow decorated in an eclectic art deco style. She loves cooking and inviting friends over for authentic Italian meals, invigorating conversations and watching movies from her classic collection. She volunteers for *A Girl's World,* a local program empowering elementary school girls to think globally. Ava and her husband enjoy speed walking in their neighborhood. Shopping for one-of-a-kind fashion pieces at vintage stores and scouring up-scale antique shops and flea markets for art deco objects are Ava's hobbies. *Check out Ava's personification and look at the necessary information it takes to design, create and perfect an empowering image which also maintains her authenticity.*

Ava's Personification

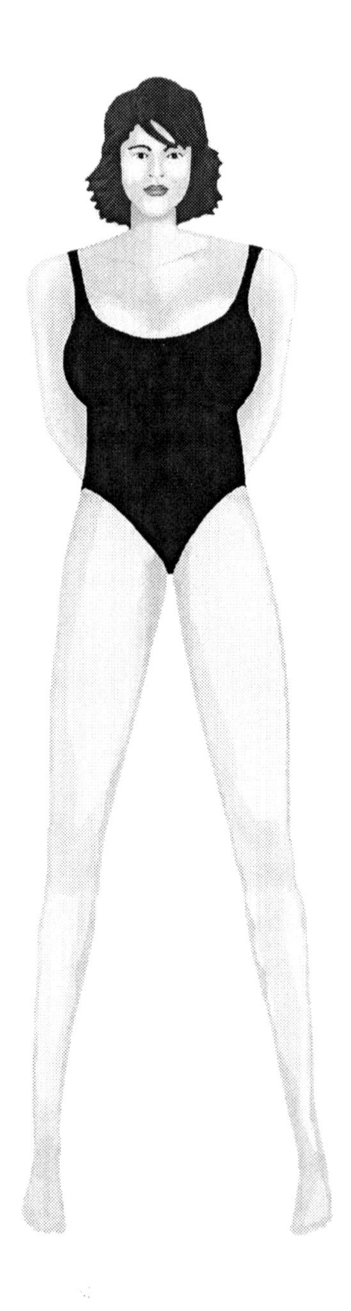

Age Height Weight

28 5'7" 147

Size Frame

10 Medium

Body Type Body Shape

Mesomorphic Inverted Pear

Challenge

Camouflaging a short torso and minimizing a full bust

Career Choice

Film and Video Editor

Lifestyle

Ava is a married in-town eclectic who collects classic movies and art deco. She is healthy and fit and loves cooking and entertaining at home.

Fashion Personality Type

Glamorous and Classic

Color Season

Warm autumn—copper skin tone, turquoise eyes and auburn hair.

Ava in Business Casual Attire

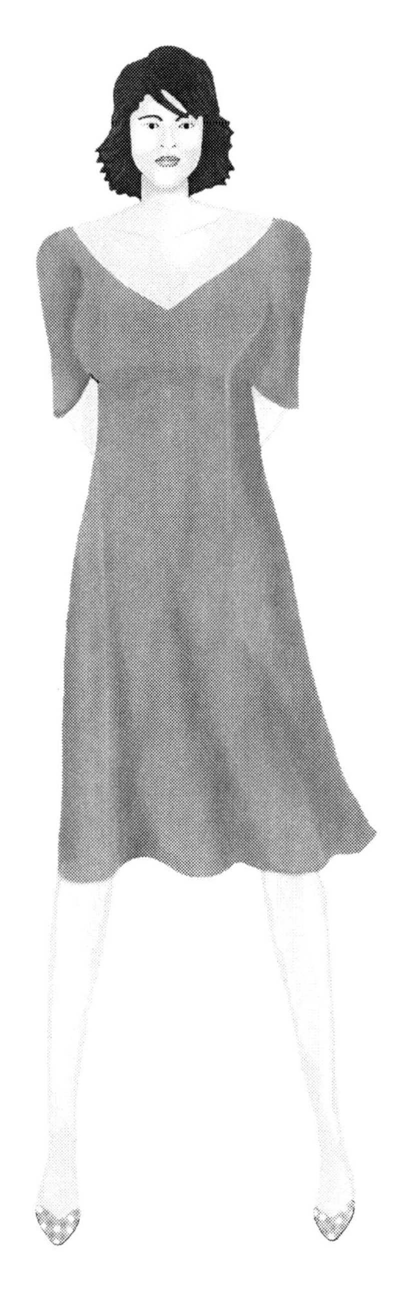

Ava loves dressing womanly and feeling glamorous every day if she has her way. However, now that she works from home seven to nine hours a day, five days a week, her glamorous work clothes are too restrictive. Nevertheless, she longs to feel glamorous in beautiful, well-fitting clothes again. Her image challenge is to balance out her wide shoulders and full bust while creating a dressed-down, easygoing glamorous look, an elegant feel that flows naturally with her living and working space at home.

1. First and foremost, Ava will want to draw attention from her waist down—and not make the mistake of wearing blouson bodice blouses, oversized shirts or thin spaghetti straps.

2. She loves femininity, but needs comfort and fluidity, so I've selected a periwinkle V-neck sweeping dress in a light-weight jersey.

3. The V-neck elongates, minimizes the bust and softens her shape.

4. The slightly cinched waist gives the illusion of a longer torso.

5. The flared princess cut adds movement and elegance that fits into Ava's fashion personality and relaxed lifestyle.

6. The dress length falls just below her knee—showing off fabulously long, elegant legs.

7. The elegant mules are easy to slide on for running errands, yet comfortable and easy to kick off for indoor ease.

This glamorous, yet relaxed look satisfies Ava's need to express her femininity while allowing her to feel relaxed and comfortable while she works from home.

Ava's Fashion and Style Checklist:

1.Golden brown 40's—style fitted worsted wool peplum blazer
2.Brown silk charmeuse fitted blouse
3.Brown boatneck long-sleeve cotton/lycra blend tee
4.Brown wide leg soft stretch cotton/lycra blend pants
5.Orange viscose keyhole halter dress with silver neck ring
6. Rust brocade pencil skirt
7.Cream draping V-neck silk chiffon tunic
8.Camel boatneck short sleeve cotton/lycra blend tee
9.Camel wide-leg soft-stretch cotton/lycra blend pants
10. Cream satin evening pants
11. White cotton button-down fitted shirt
12. White cotton elbow-length wrap shirt
13. Orange floral retro A-line boatneck dress
14. Camel cashmere zip hoodie
15. Periwinkle princess-cut V-neck jersey dress
16. Periwinkle velour sweatsuit
17. Periwinkle, pink and cream low-heel mules
18. Brown peep-toe leather and fabric heels
19. Vintage cream pearl-and-glass beaded clutch
20. Minimizing bras

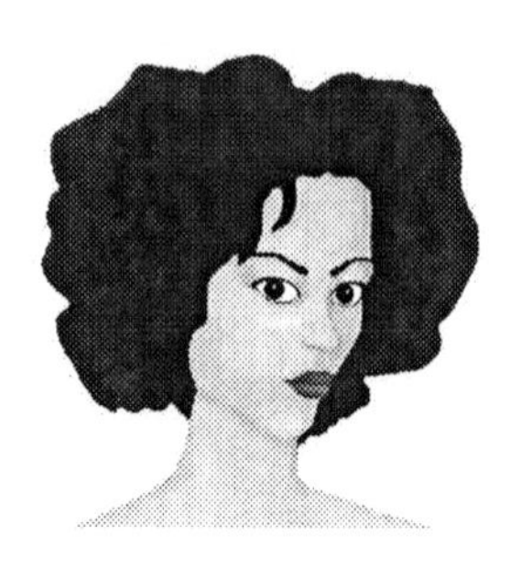

Isabella is a spirited and dramatic thirty-three-year-old entertainment attorney whose passion is empowering her clients to artistic and financial freedom. She and Tony, her husband of seven years, are a dynamic duo, teaming up as attorney and agent to protect their clients' intellectual property, to write and review contracts and to guide their careers to success. Isabella is professional, ethical, effective and efficient in her practice and in negotiating the right deals for her clients. For her, building and maintaining meaningful relationships is her first priority—for herself, her family and her clients. She loves entertaining and going to work-related events and is usually the life of the party.

Isabella and Tony, their-three-year-old daughter, Samantha, and two cocker spaniels, Max and Mindy, live in the suburbs in an elaborately decorated but comfortable Mediterranean Revival—style home. She is committed to a four-day work week and reserving every Monday for mother-daughter play dates. Her image challenge is her endomorphic apple shape and dressing too flamboyantly. However, she is learning to camouflage her substantial waistline and to accentuate her beautiful, expressive eyes and shapely legs. She maintains optimal health and watches her mid-section, which is prone to store fat, by playing tennis, swimming, following a balanced Mediterranean diet and making a point to connect with her best girlfriends twice a year at holistic retreats and spas. Isabella provides pro bono legal services at Assistant Lawyers for the Arts and serves as a legal consultant for the Spanish Writers Export Office. She speaks English, Spanish, French and Italian fluently. Her all-time favorite thing in the world is the Christmas holiday season and spending it with her large extended family. *Check out Isabella's personification and consider what it takes to design, create and perfect an empowering image for her that maintains her authenticity.*

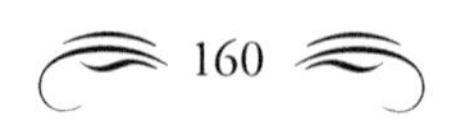

Isabella's Personification

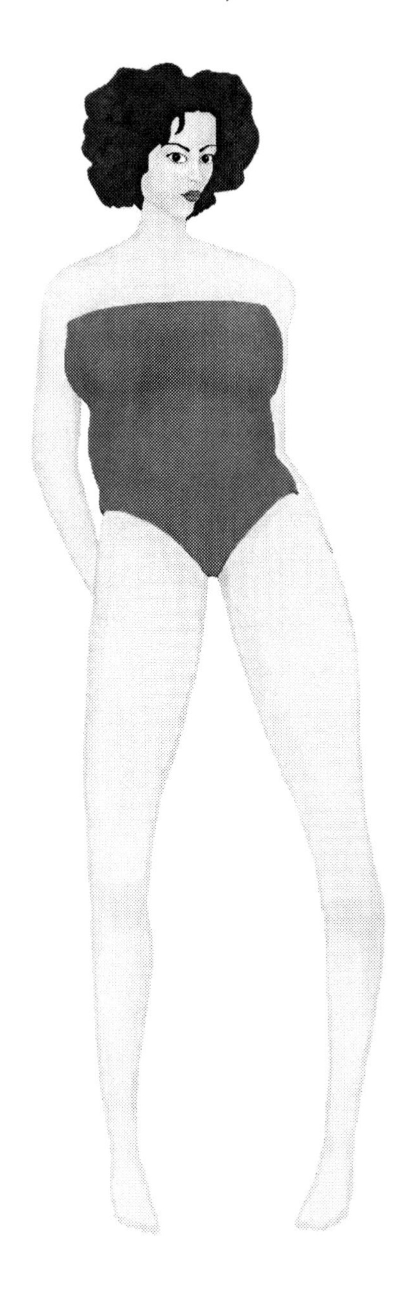

Age Height Weight

33 5'5" 145

Size Frame

10/12 Medium

Body Type Body Shape

Endomorphic Apple

Challenge

Thick-waisted and round abdomen

Career Choice

Entertainment Attorney

Lifestyle

Isabella is married with one child. She lives a Suburban Mediterranean lifestyle. Isabella loves closing the right deals for her clients and going on retreats with her husband to celebrate.

Fashion Personality Type

Avant Garde and Dramatic

Color Season

Cool winter—dark olive skin tone, dark brown eyes and brown hair.

Isabella in Power Business Attire

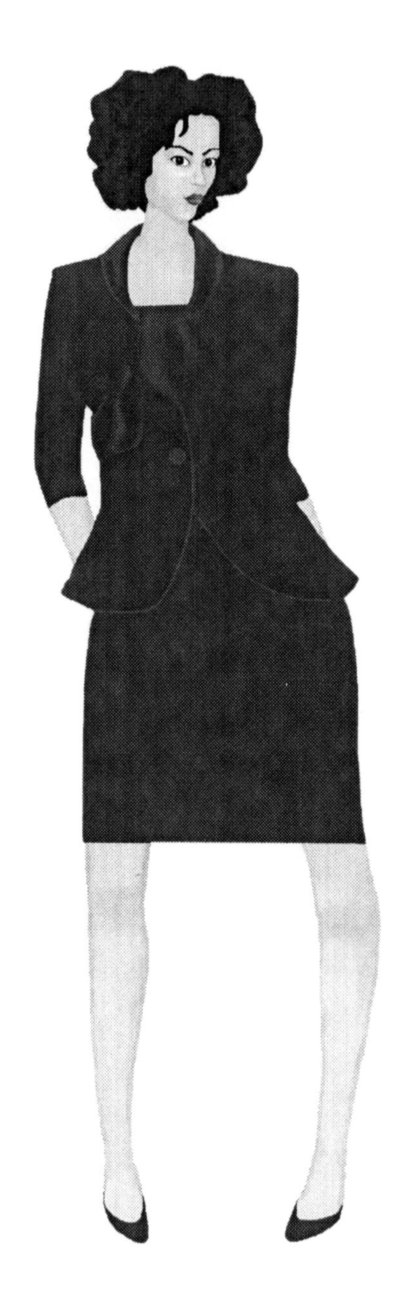

Striking and colorful, Isabella hardly ever needs an introduction. Her personality attracts others to her in a positive way. She loves fashion and always wanted to be a high-fashion model, but realized at age eighteen that she would probably never grow past her current height of five feet and five inches—she determined she would become an attorney instead. Her image challenge is her thick, rounded abdomen and understanding how to camouflage her thick waistline in order to incorporate selected pieces of high-fashion clothes into her wardrobe.

1.First and foremost, Isabella will want to avoid boxy, shapeless clothes, clingy fabrics and thin belts that draw attention to her waist. She can look fabulous with shapely, well-tailored separates and outfits.

2. She loves expensive designer clothes in bold colors, so I've selected a deep sapphire, well-tailored sleeveless, empire waist dress and sharp jacket in silk.

3. This silhouette adds the illusion of curves and the color adds the drama that she loves.

4. The low, open neck of the dress and jacket softens and elongates her short, thick neck.

5. The empire waist of the dress flares out slightly, just below the bust and hides her thick waist and round tummy if she wants to remove her jacket.

6. The shoulders of the jacket are softly padded to square and balance her shape.

7. The elbow-length fitted sleeves elongate.

8. The gently cinched waist gives the illusion of a leaner waistline.

9. The 40's style fitted jacket accommodates Isabella's breasts and add curves and elegance.

10. The knee-length pencil skirt shows off Isabella's great legs.

11. The sapphire stiletto pumps add height and elegance.

This well-fitted designer look is perfect for Isabella's busy and flamboyant lifestyle of business dinners, entertaining and events. The deep sapphire indulges her need to be bold without complicating the monochromatic look of the two-piece ensemble.

Isabella's Fashion and Style Checklist:

1.Sapphire empire waist dress with tailored jacket
2.Black classic light-weight wool suit with tailored cinched waist jacket and pencil skirt
3.Black polished pin-striped tailored skirt suit with red threads
4.Black silky satin empire waist camisole
5.Black boot-cut jeans
6.Black wide-leg silk evening pants
7.Red designer silk and wool blend pencil skirt suit trimmed in beige and brown
8.Red silk evening pantsuit with one-button jacket and flared cuffless pant
9.White classic cotton fitted cuffed blouse
10. White cotton pique structured jacket and pencil skirt ensemble
11. Cream boat neck silk charmeuse top
12. Cream wide V-neck empire waist satin tunic
13. Shocking pink wide V-neck, sleeveless, empire waist evening top
14. Black jewel-encrusted leather mules with three-inch heel
15. Brown fabric peep-toe with red accents and three-inch heel
16. Red sexy and sassy three-inch strappy sandals
17. Diamond studs
18. Black crocodile briefcase
19. Nude torso waist shaper
20. Minimizing bras

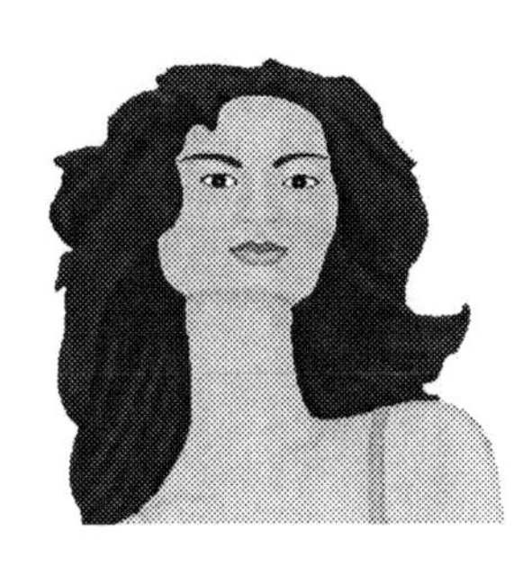

Angela is a thirty-nine-year-old divorced mother of two daughters, Tia, age eight, and Tara, age six. She always knew she would become a doctor and contribute her fair share to the world. Respected and admired by her peers and colleagues, Angela is a board-certified radiologist at an inner-city hospital specializing in body imaging. After twenty-six years of school, four years of being a full-time stay-at-home mom, followed by an additional one-year fellowship, she landed her dream job and has not looked back. She loves staying on top of her skills while experiencing the spirit and lifestyle of fabulous cities for six to twelve weeks of fellowship work during the summer months.

Angela grew up with a passion for fashion and style and loves looking fabulous, even wearing a white lab coat. However, her image challenge has been dressing less flirtatiously at work while maintaining her authentic feminine side and balancing her pear-shaped body. She and her girls live in a suburban manor home, decorated in a comfortable modern style with lots of open space for the girls and their friends. Her home is peaceful and always stocked with quick, healthy snacks, simple meals and bottled water. They also love eating out, taking forty-minute drives to visit Angela's parents and indulging in wonderful home-cooked meals. Angela and her daughters love it when girlfriends visit and sleepover. She also enjoys going to movies and riding bikes in their neighborhood with Tia and Tara. Angela is a member of the American College of Radiology and is committed to giving her time and efforts to community service work as a member of *Links, Incorporated* a non-profit community service organization. *Check out Angela's personification and the essentials it takes to design, create and perfect an empowering image for her that upholds authenticity.*

Angela's Personification

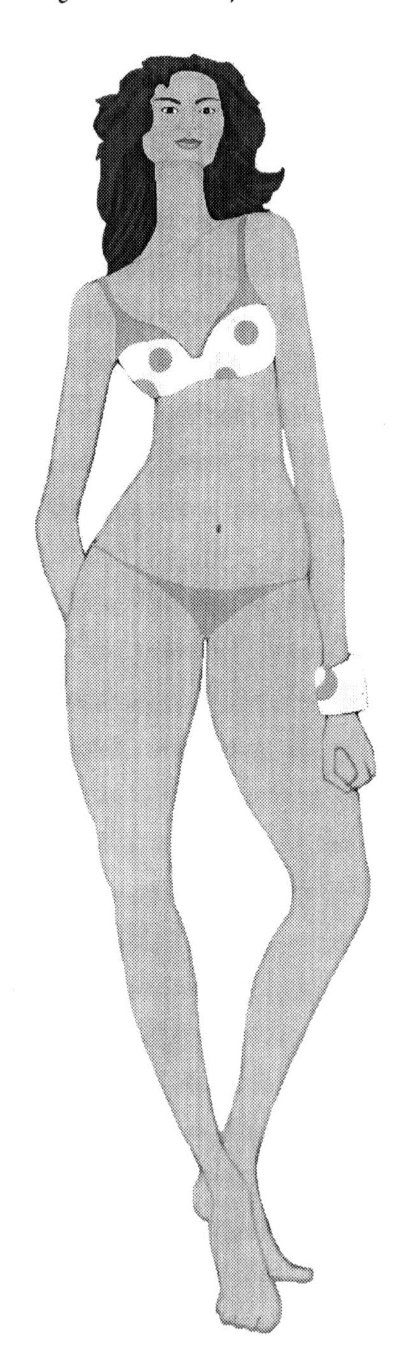

Age Height Weight

39 5'4" 135

Size Frame

6/8 Medium

Body Type Body Shape

Ectomorphic Pear

Challenge

Balancing her top and bottom and not dressing too seductively for work.

Career Choice

Radiologist

Lifestyle

Angela is a healthy and fit divorced, suburban, modernist and mother of two. She is intellectually stimulating and loves spending time with her daughters and being at the top in her work.

Fashion Personality Type

Flirtatious and Glamorous

Color Season

Warm autumn—caramel skin tone, brown eyes and golden brown hair.

Angela in Business Casual Attire

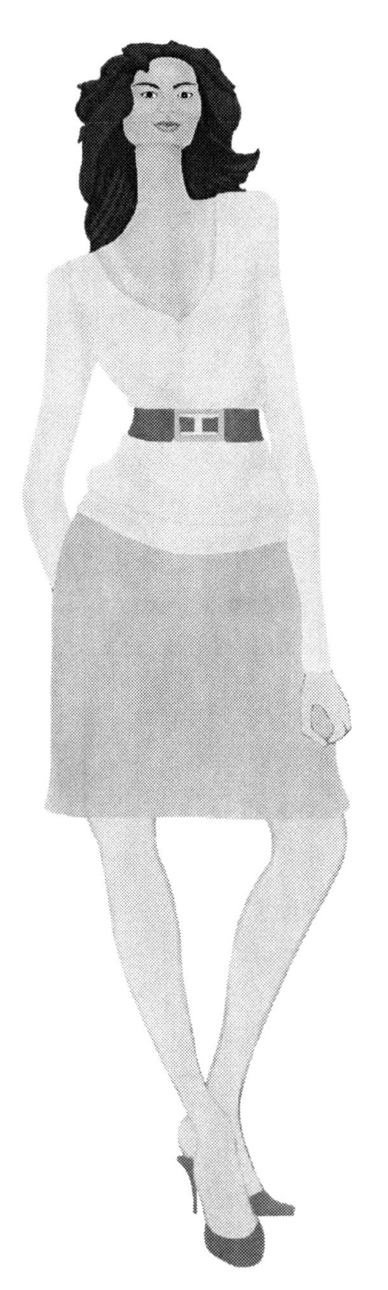

Angela's flirtatious personality type is authentic and attractive. However, her image challenge has been that she dresses too alluringly for her work at an inner-city hospital. As a board-certified radiologist it is important that she maintains a certain level of professionalism, but at the same time she wants to project her authentic feminine side. The goal is to balance her pear-shaped body proportionally, and professionally, while keeping it somewhat girlie.

1. First and foremost, Angela will want to balance her top with her bottom by adding more volume on top and by avoiding anything that draws attention to her hips and thighs. The most effective way to accomplish this is to dress her in separates to control fit.

2. She loves easy-flowing fabrics that wrap and float around her body, so I've chosen to mix and match a cozy combination of cashmere, flowing silk chiffon and seasonally worsted wool.

3.The long-sleeved, loose-fitting coral cashmere sweater has a wide, draped collar that accentuates Angela's beautiful neck.

4.The shoulders are softly padded to add volume—balancing out her shoulders and hips.

5.The elegant silk chiffon light coral blouse peaks out just enough for coverage and adds another exquisite texture.

6.The sweater length stops just below the waist.

7.The darker-colored light orange A-line skirt in lightweight wool beautifully accommodates Angela's full hips and thighs and falls at the knee.

8.The brown croc belt accentuates Angela's overall silhouette.

9.The brown croc classic high-heel sling-backs are womanly.

This feminine, soft and elegant look is just what the doctor ordered for Angela. From under her white lab coat—you'll hardly notice it, but when the coat comes off, the flirtatious girly side comes out.

Angela's Fashion and Style Checklist:

1. Chocolate three-piece classic suit in light-weight wool—structured jacket with cinched waist, A-line skirt and flared pants
2. Brown super-soft suede military-inspired jacket
3. Brown A-line light-weight wool skirt
4. Brown cotton elegant wide-leg pants
5. Coral wide V-neck cashmere sweater
6. Coral silk chiffon frilly blouse
7. Soft orange A-line worsted wool skirt
8. Cream light-weight wool single-button structured jacket
9. Cream silk chiffon camisole
10. Cream short sleeve boatneck silk tee
11. Dark-wash mid-rise jeans
12. Kelly green velour sweatsuit
13. Golden brown V-neck belted waist double crepe dress
14. Sand leather kitten-heel slides
15. Brown crocodile classic sling-backs
16. Diamond drop earrings
17. Platinum-and-gold watch
18. Brown crocodile designer buckle bag
19. Enhancing bras
20. Detachable shoulder pads

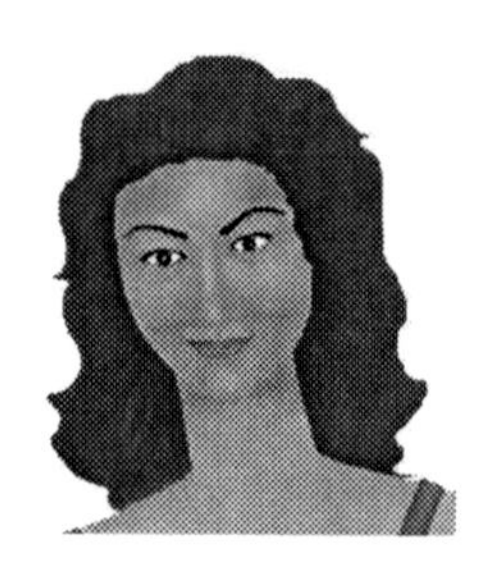

Hannah is a forty-eight-year-old special education teacher who is committed to the learning process of her middle-school students. She received a national education award for developing the most progressive and cutting-edge Individual Education Program for her students for two consecutive years. But what Hannah is especially proud of is combining her love for special-needs children with her love and passion for horses—providing safe and fun experiences for children and their parents on weekends and holidays. She and Joe, her husband of twenty-eight years, left the suburbs after their sons, Victor, Michael and Robert graduated from high school, buying a farm house and property an hour and a half from the city. Hannah gives displaced non-competitive racehorses a home and her students a place to let go, have fun, go on trail rides and learn about horses. She and her husband live in a ranch-style home, decorated in a traditional rustic style. There is always someone at Hannah's home, especially at her kitchen table—neighbors talking or eating, her husband making arrangements for one of their college boys or Hannah scheduling kids for trail riding.

Hannah and her husband share a wholesome and simple lifestyle. She has always maintained her weight with natural workouts through horseback riding, playing basketball with her boys and coaching the girls' volley ball team at her middle-school. Hannah is 6'2" and has a beautifully toned hourglass body. Her image challenge is finding fashions that are long enough for her and fit her small waist. She also wants to dress more feminine for special occasions.

Hannah relaxes by working in her garden. She shares the vegetables with the teachers at her school and her city friends, whom she and Joe meet in the city on Thursdays for cocktails, dinner and comedy. *Check out Hannah's personification and the vital information it takes to design, create and perfect an empowering image which asserts her authenticity.*

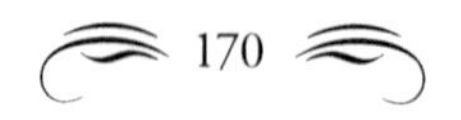

Hannah's Personification

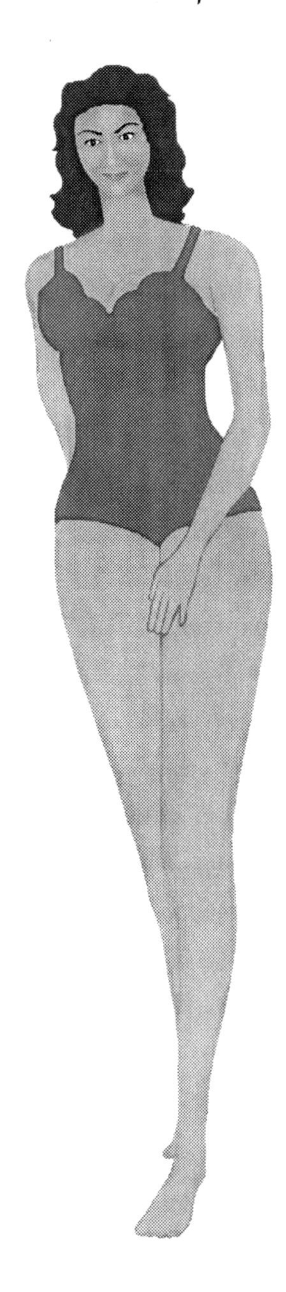

Age Height Weight

48 6'2" 170

Size Frame

14/16 Large

Body Type Body Shape

Mesomorphic Hourglass

Challenge

Find fashionable feminine clothes that fit properly

Career Choice

Special Education Teacher

Lifestyle

Hannah is married with three college-age sons; she maintains a traditional rural lifestyle; she loves children and horses and is active, healthy and fit.

Fashion Personality Type

Casual and Western

Color Season

Cool winter—dark brown skin tone, dark brown eyes and black hair.

Hannah in Dressy Casual Attire:

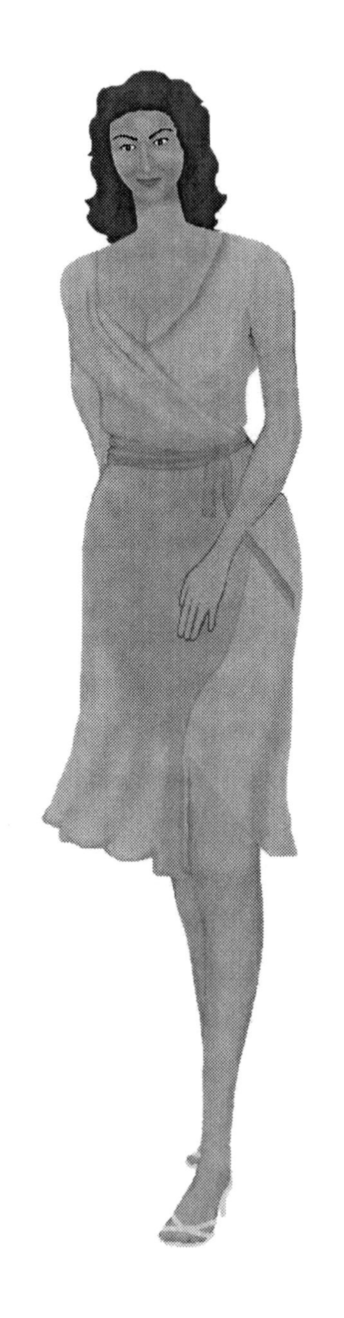

Hannah's gorgeous six-feet-two-inch frame is a knock-out! For the past fifteen years she has worn only active casual and Western wear, limited by her size and height. Her dressed-down super-casual look also worked for Hannah as a middle-school special-education teacher. Her image challenge is finding more feminine fashions for special occasions that fit her fabulous hourglass figure.

1.First and foremost, Hannah will want to stay away from halter tops, capped sleeves, spaghetti straps, super-size tee-shirts, chunky knits and anything that makes her look like she is being smothered by her breasts.

2.Hannah is now ready to put forth the effort in re-vamping her womanly side, so I've chosen a very simple yet elegant soft pink wrap dress with layers and layers of silk chiffon.

3. The plunging V-neckline enhances and lengthens her décolletage and sets the stage for feminine elegance.
4. The crisscross effects of the wrap dress lifts and separates while accentuating the waist.
5. The icy pink, softly flared bias-cut dress makes Hannah's top look smaller.
6. Her nude legs and strappy, sexy sandals complete her look.

The simplicity of this elegant dress is perfect for Hannah and the icy pink color is fabulous against her dark skin tone. All she has to do is slip into the dress and go, which alleviates her fears of *getting ready.*

Hannah's Fashion and Style Checklist:

1.Icy blue high sheen cotton belted jacket with silver hardware
2.Navy wide boatneck bell-sleeve cotton/lycra blend tee
3.Navy light-weight wool flat front-flared cuffed pants
4.Black long-sleeve V-neck silk tee
5.Black flat front boot-cut cuffed wool trousers
6.Black long-sleeve double crepe wrap dress
7.Dark wash boot-cut jeans with a not-too-high rise
8.Faded boot-cut jeans with a not-too-high rise
9.Camel suede double-breasted tailored jacket
10. White three-quarter-length cotton wrap blouse
11. Pink wide boatneck bell-sleeve cotton/lycra blend tee
12. Cream long-sleeve light-weight wool V-neck twin set
13. Icy pink silk chiffon and satin wrap dress
14. Cracked silver kitten-heel slides
15. Silver "Walking Liberty Half Dollar" belt
16. Silver horse drop earrings and silver watch
17. Black classic sling-backs with two and a half inch heel
18. Brown alligator cowboy boots
19. Brown leather bucket bag
20. Support bras

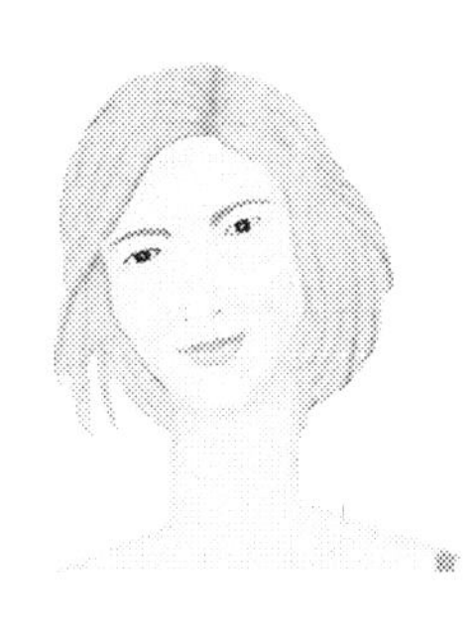

Rebecca is a fifty-seven-year-old single mother of one daughter, twenty-six-year-old Lynn. She is the author of fifteen books and has won the National Book Award for *When Being Feminine Was In,* a collection of short stories and is the founder of The Universal Creative Writer's Network, a non-profit, volunteer-based organization created by writers for writers.

Rebecca lives alone in a downtown high-rise condominium, decorated in a sophisticated modern style. She travels frequently for book signings and speaking engagements and rarely cooks—preferring to have delicious and nutritious meals delivered to her home. That is, when she is not eating out with her daughter, having lunch with her girlfriends or attending one of her many social functions, where she is often asked to chair or participate in some benevolent way. Rebecca knows she is blessed with her balanced body and high metabolism and can wear almost anything. She stays in shape by swimming as often as she can, eating balanced portions of whatever she likes and moderate alcohol consumption. Her image challenge is to incorporate color into her wardrobe which, for the last fifteen years, has been completely monochromatic and dominated by pastels.

Rebecca appreciates being admired for her writing and her professionalism and also being part of the social scene, but her favorite place to be is in her own home, curled up watching *I Love Lucy* reruns or on the phone with one of her four sisters. She and her daughter, along with her sisters, share a two-week beauty and spiritual retreat every August in Arizona. They leave cell phones, laptops and wireless devices at home. *Check out her personification and the essentials it takes to design, create and perfect an empowering image for her that heightens her authenticity.*

Rebecca's Personification

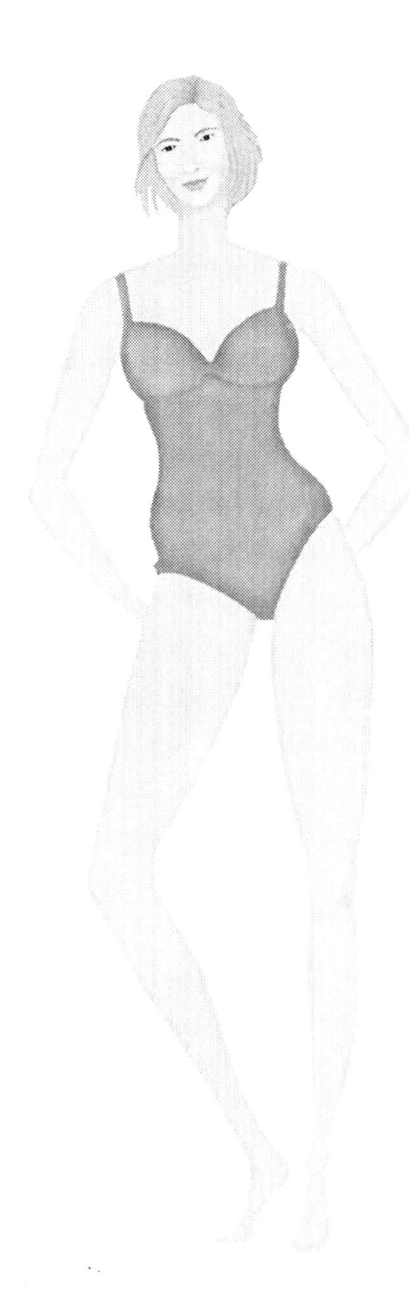

Age Height Weight

57 5'9" 140

Size Frame

6/8 Small

Body Type Body Shape

Ectomorphic Balanced

Challenge

Incorporating color into an existing monochromatic wardrobe

Career Choice

Novelist

Lifestyle

Rebecca is a single, urban modernist with one adult daughter. She loves quiet days, swimming and lying by the pool, reading and lunching with her daughter.

Fashion Personality Type

Classic and Glamorous

Color Season

Warm spring—ivory skin tone, hazel eyes and strawberry blond hair.

Rebecca in Dressy Casual Attire:

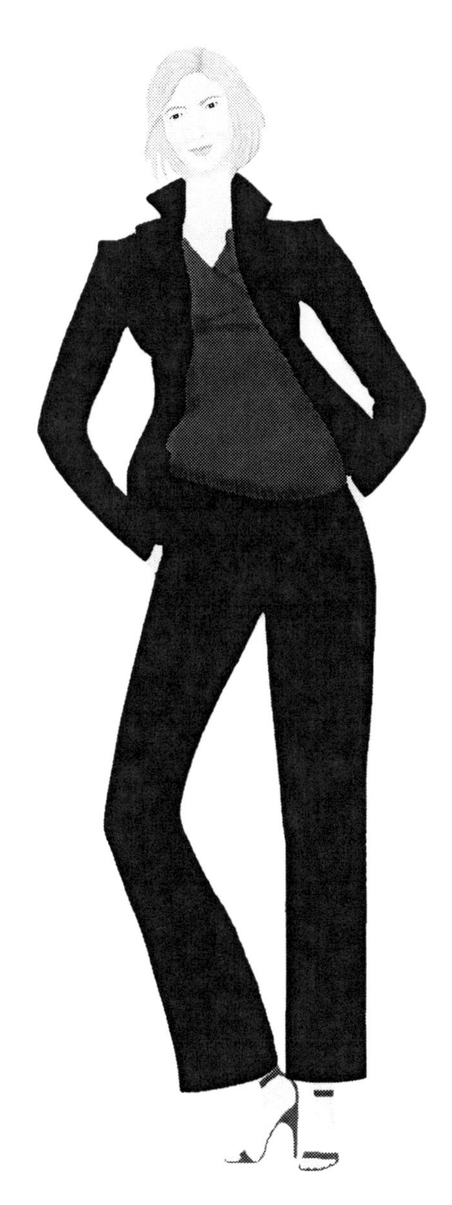

Rebecca's balanced body is easy to dress; almost everything looks good on her, with her long, lean and proportionate shape. She has a phenomenal wardrobe except that it has no color. Her image challenge is to spice up her pastel, monochromatic look.

1.First and foremost, Rebecca intends to slowly incorporate pieces with vibrant color into her existing wardrobe.

2.Rebecca loves dressing monochromatically (wearing the same color from head to toe), which is fine. However, her wardrobe colors consist of: white, cream, beige, tan, coral, peach, pink, and grey. I've chosen to compromise by agreeing with her elegant monochromatic style, but completely going for the color gusto by getting her into richer colors.

3. The elegant golden brown silk dupioni pants suit is classic and comfortable.
4. The soft brown V-neck silk and cashmere blend top is luxuriously comfortable.
5. The high-heel brown ankle strap sandals pull together a perfectly put-together look.

The golden-brown, monochromatic outfit is quite bold for Rebecca, but feeling confident after all of the positive responses and compliments she has received from others, she has chosen to add a few more colors to her existing wardrobe.

Rebecca's Fashion and Style Checklist:

1.Golden-brown high-sheen cotton-belted jacket with antique brass hardware
2.Brown, gold and cream bouclé three-quarter-length sleeve jacket and pencil skirt suit
3.Soft blue long-sleeve double crepe wrap dress
4.Golden brown silk dupioni pantsuit
5.Golden brown V-neck silk and cashmere blend sweater
6.Ivory long-sleeve silk charmeuse blouse
7.Spring blue velour sweatsuit
8.Ivory sleeveless silk turtleneck sweater
9.Champagne full-length dolman sleeve silk charmeuse lounge dress
10. Golden brown silk twin sweater set
11. Soft blue cotton piqué cuffed elbow-length wrap shirt and pencil skirt ensemble
12. Leaf green cotton/lycra blend flared pants
13. Leaf green cotton/lycra blend empire waist tunic
14. Diamond drop earrings and platinum watch
15. Champagne *peau de soie* kitten-heel mules
16. Two-toned classic pumps with three-inch heel
17. Golden brown ankle strap sandals with four-inch heel
18. Golden brown Crocodile designer bag
19. Champagne silk and mesh evening bag
20. Ivory year-round trench coat with removal lining

Getting Ready Chloé-Style

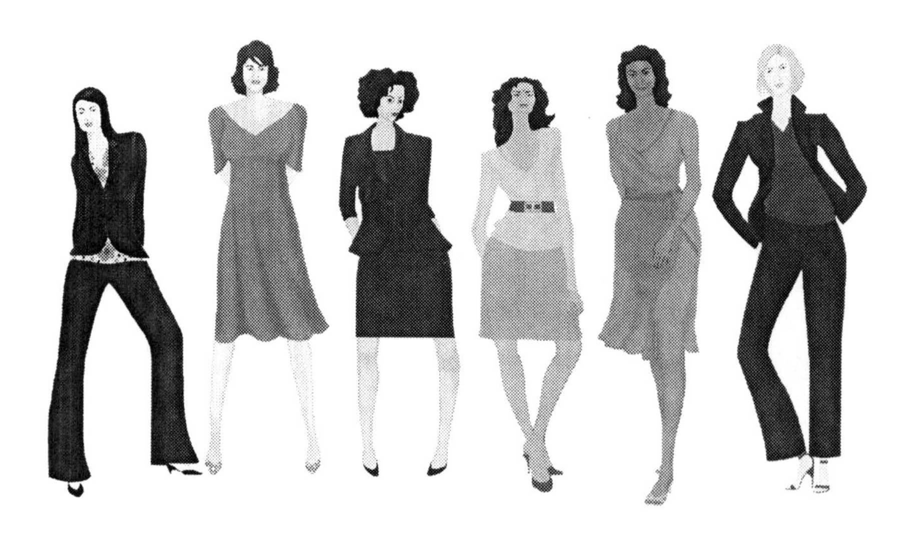

Perfecting Your Authentic Image

Managing and Maintaining Your Image

After putting in the necessary work to create your authentic image, you'll want to create a strategic plan to maintain it. Keep this in mind throughout the entire process:

- No matter what society or the media tries to dictate about your body, body image and beauty, you *must* understand that it's all superficial—it's not real.
- If you choose to embrace the uniqueness of your body, your personality and the individuality of your being, you'll have incredible personal power.
- If you determine that you are going to *be* your best self—your genuine, real self in all that you *do,* you'll increase your personal power.
- If you determine *your ideal*, and set daily goals to reach it, let it become your way of life, your lifestyle and your work, you'll increase your personal power and empower the world.
- If you enhance or design your personal image to harmonize with your ideal and who you want to be in the world, always connected honestly and harmoniously with your body type and shape, you'll *perfect your authentic image.*

My goal is to sell you on yourself so that you *can* perfect your authentic image and project it to the world. Your good looks and polished image will need an effective and efficient maintenance plan that starts right where you are.

Note: If you are a weight-problem person, do one of two things: commit right now to follow a wellness program and get support—or accept and love the body that you have and learn how to dress fabulously for your body type and shape. If you suffer from anorexia, bulimia, obesity or any eating disorder please contact the National Eating Disorder Association (NEDA) by calling 800.931.2237 or 206.382.3587 or going online at info@nationaleatingdisorders.org. You may also contact the Eating Disorder Information Network (EDIN) by calling 404.816.3346 or visit online at www.edin-ga.org, or the American Obesity Association (AOA) by calling 202.776.7711 or go online at www.obesity.org.

Maintaining Image Power

- Eat properly by including lots of fresh live foods in your daily diet.
- Drink lots of water.
- Follow a wellness program and get your beauty rest.
- Keep your teeth clean and white.
- Smile big.
- Laugh out loud—often.
- Learn how to apply beautiful, natural-looking make-up—quick.
- Keep a haircut and style that will minimize bad hair days.
- Keep cute, natural-looking hair pieces, wigs and/or hair accessories if you're prone to having too many bad hair days even with a great cut and style.
- Maintain a pleasing personality—it will attract others to you in a positive way.

- Take care of your body and dress like you are proud of it (this does not mean exposing your body in any way less than a lady would).
- Maintain your wardrobe by keeping your closet organized and clutter-free.

Self-Love and Acceptance

- After you bathe or shower—stand in front of your full-length mirror—nude.
- Look at yourself lovingly as you affirm the positive traits of your body and each of its parts—create your own positive daily affirmations.
- Put your favorite music on and continue to admire your body in the mirror as you dance.
- Feel the love that God has poured into your body as you moisturize and caress it with your favorite lotions and oils.
- You will begin to acquire an amazing understanding of your own authenticity.
- Your body language will be positive and powerful.
- You will set measurable and achievable goals for all areas of your life.
- You will make a strategic plan to accomplish your goals.
- You will love and respect yourself and your body.
- You will strive to be your most excellent self.
- You will feel and look absolutely amazing.

Answer These Questions

1.What excuses have I used in the past to stop me from looking consistently great? *List them.*

2.Do I understand that my image could be one of my most powerful tools? *Explain.*

3.How can I take advantage of my attributes? *Make a list.*

4.What do I want to communicate about myself? *Make a list.*

5.What do I need to do today to create and perfect my authentic image? *Make your to-do list.*

Creating Your Thirty-Day Image Improvement Plan

Now that you understand all the necessary steps to creating and perfecting your authentic image, I want you to create a thirty-day image improvement plan that states:

Between now and thirty days from today, I will break these habits:

1.Negative thinking and language about my body.

2.Obsessing about the sizes that I wear.

3.Gossiping about another woman's look behind her back. The more I can appreciate other women's beauty and body image, the more I can appreciate my own.

Between now and thirty days from today I will acquire these habits:

1.Giving my body the attention it deserves.

2.Refining my poise and posture and the way that I walk.

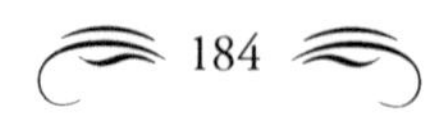

3. Focusing more on my assets.

4. Loving myself, as ***I am*** and who ***I am***.

Between now and thirty days from today I will sharpen my image in these ways:

1. Get a great haircut and style. It is essential to my overall image.

2. Enhance my looks with the right skin-care regime and the right cosmetics.

3. Invest in quality fabrics and quality shoes.

4. Examine my appearance each morning. Ask myself, "What am I projecting?"

5. Be articulate and well informed.

6. Enjoy the most beautiful gift of all, the sound of laughter.

7. Put a time limit on when I will achieve my goals. *This will help you to stay focused.*

8. Make an appointment to meet and work with an Image Coach, if necessary. You may contact Total Image Enhancement at 404.256.4228 or, online at www.totalimageenhancement.com.

Afterword

Now that you understand how body image, self-esteem and fashion are all intertwined, I want you to use this information to empower yourself, to take control of your image, and present your authentic self to the world. I want you to begin living your life to the fullest each day and to take advantage of every chance to make life rewarding and pleasurable.

When you wake up in the morning, express in your own way how much you love and honor God, and the wonder and beauty of life. Thank your body for holding you up and getting you where you want to go. I want you to start each day by looking into the mirror and smiling back at yourself. Remember, what you project in the mirror is what you'll always get back in return. Tell yourself how much *you* like *you* and what you're going to do for yourself this day. Tell yourself that you love being true to yourself, and that you're going to enjoy the process of creating, developing and maintaining your authentic image. Use kind and beautiful words and phrases when referring to yourself and your body. Always be proud of who you are, yet always strive to be just a little bit better. That way you are always getting just a little bit better and on top of your plan.

If there is something about your body that you want to work on, tell your body how you're going to take care of it because you love it so much. Let your body know that you understand that it is genuine and unique and that you are very aware that God created only one. As you dress yourself, remember the *Selfing Process* and allow yourself to *put on* all while being perfectly *you*. When you're Getting Ready Chloé-Style, it does not matter if you're putting on for work, for fun, for a glamorous evening out, or for your favorite sport—you will remain true to yourself and to your authentic image. And when you step out into the world to take on the day, the job, the fun, the event, and all of life, you will be poised, polished, and perfectly put together—a true Inner Beauty Being!

Enjoy your authenticity!

About the Author

Chloé Taylor Brown is the president and chief image officer of Total Image Enhancement, a privately held consulting firm offering a variety of image development programs that assist corporations, organizations and professionals in creating, perfecting and managing their personal, professional and corporate image. Chloé is a speaker and seminar leader, specializing in image management and body image esteem. She speaks to thousands of women annually, utilizing her positive and proven ***"Selfing Process"*** to illustrate that looking your very best is much more than wearing a designer suit. Chloé combines personal experiences with proven techniques to deliver powerful presentations that explain in practical terms how to project inner beauty to the world in a completely authentic way.

This former international fashion model has over twenty combined years in the fashion and image industries. Her message is that a polished and trustworthy appearance can be created and perfected for anyone—individuals of all ages and interests, including career climbers, soccer moms, artists, business owners and big dreamers—and she outlines how to do so while captivating her audiences with funny, original stories. Chloé lives in Atlanta, Georgia, with her husband Rick and children, Jade, Taylor and Joshua.

Fashion and Image Word List

A

Aesthetician: A person who specializes in the study of skin care.

A–line: A skirt or dress shape that kicks out from the bust or waist to make an 'A' shape silhouette.

Argyle: A knitted design of solid diamond blocks contrasted in a pattern, often used for socks and jumpers.

Asymmetric: Uneven or one-sided; diagonal hemlines; one-shouldered tops, strap or sleeve.

Authentic: Being trustworthy, reliable, genuine, legitimate, original, real and true.

B

Balance Line: A horizontal or vertical line from which the pluses and minuses of a figure shape are evaluated.

Bateau: A neckline that follows the curve of the collarbone, sometimes called boatneck.

Batwing: A long, broad sleeve shape made from a large triangular piece of fabric from the shoulder to the wrist, then joining wrist to waist, very popular in the 1980's.

Bell Sleeve: A sleeve that is full and flares out at the lower edge like a bell.

Bias Cut: Cutting fabric diagonally across the grain, causing the material to drape fluidly and elegantly across the body. Often used for silk or satin dresses for maximum slink factor.

Bishop Sleeve: A sleeve that is full in the lower part and held by a band at the wrist.

Blazer: A lightweight, loose-fitting sports jacket, often striped or worn as part of a uniform, usually worn below the hip.

Blouson: A gathered bodice bloused to give the effect of fullness and gathered in at the waist.

Bodice: The part of the garment above the waist.

Body Awareness: Understanding, loving and accepting your body for its authenticity while being conscious of what it can and cannot do.

Body Suit: An all-in-one that's close-fitting as to appear to be second skin.

Bomber Jacket: A sporty waist-length cropped jacket with a rounded or puffed-out body with zip fastening from waist to neck.

Bouclé: ("boo clay"). Woven or knitted fabric with looped or knotted texture.

Box Pleat: A pleat made of two flat folds turned inward towards each other, creating a boxlike shape on the front of the garment.

Brocade: A rich, Jacquard weave fabric with a woven design of raised figures and floral motifs—pattern emphasized by contrast in weave or colors.

C

Cable Knit: Knit in a raised loop stripe resembling a twisted cable, used in knitted sweaters.

Camisole: A sleeveless lingerie-like outer garment worn as a blouse under a jacket.

Cap Sleeve: A short sleeve just covering the shoulder that does not continue under the arm.

Cape: A sleeveless outergarment that hangs loose from the shoulders, covering the arms and back.

Capri Pants: Loose pants slightly tapered to the mid-calf.

Cardigan: A close-fitting collarless sweater or jacket with a front-center closing.

Cat Suit: An all-in-one garment usually zipped or buttoned from navel to neck.

***Chamber á coucher*:** French—a bedroom.

Chain Mail: A flexible and luxurious fabric of many interwoven metal rings used in suits of armor. Similar version is *metal mesh.*

Chemise: An undergarment or dress styled like a long undershirt or loose slip.

Chenille: Silk, rayon, cotton or wool combined and tufted, creating a soft luxurious velvet-like pile.

Chesterfield: A plain coat that usually has a velvet-notched collar.

Chevron: V-shape stripes.

Cigarette Pants: Very narrow-fitting trousers that taper towards the ankle.

Coat Dress: A dress that has coat-like lines with a front closing.

Cocktail Dress: A short, knee-length dress usually of a lightweight wool, satin, silk or velvet fabric. Often cut to reveal the shoulders and arms.

***Confulma*:** Confusion and drama.

Contrast: Distinct differences in color, shading, fabric, etc.

Corset: A flattering one-piece lingerie item—a bra and panty-girdle in one that is body-shaping.

Cowl: A soft draping of fabric, cut so that the fabric can hang in soft folds. Often found on necklines, backs and even trousers.

Crepe: Thin, gauzy, silk fabric usually crinkled in some way.

Crew: A rounded neckline that hugs the throat.

Culottes: Informal trouser-like garment with wide cropped legs giving the illusion of a full skirt.

Cummerbund: A wide cloth worn as a waist sash.

Cutout: An actual cut out of fabric from a garment in a controlled fashion.

D

Décolleté: A very low neckline which exposes either the back or the cleavage of the bosom; traditionally worn on ball gowns and evening wear.

Detail Line: A line that minimizes or maximizes a figure and a style line (hemlines, trims, small accessories, fabric texture and prints).

Design Line: A line that can add height, width, length, and curves to a figure or the contour of a body; also called a figure line.

Dolman: A sleeve that is set into a deep armhole; resembles a kimono sleeve.

Draping: A technique of hanging fabric in folds; in draped garments, hemlines are often uneven.

Double-Breasted: A front closing which overlaps enough to allow for two rows of buttons.

E

Empire Cut: A dress or gown with a high waistline (décolleté) and a straight skirt, popular with ladies of the 17th century.

Ensemble: An entire outfit.

Epaulet: A shoulder trimming; usually a band secured by a button.

Essential Nutrients: Carbohydrates, fats, proteins, minerals, vitamins and water.

F

Fashion: The prevailing style or mode in dressing.

Fatigues: Military combat apparel.

Fishnet: Open-weave knit, more often associated with hosiery, which became a defining feature of Punk dress in the late 1970s.

Fishtail: A fan-shaped addition to the train of a dress, popular in evening gowns; a fish-like train that follows behind the wearer.

Flannel: A towel-like short pile fabric popular for sportswear.

Flare: A part of a garment that widens or spreads out.

Fluted: A long sleeve flared at the wrist.

Funnel Collar: A large over collar that stands away from the neck. Similar to the turtle neck but larger.

G

Gore: A tapered section of a garment, wider at the lower edge.

H

Halter Neck: A dress or top shape with a high panel on the front, which is then tied around the neck, exposing the back and shoulders.

Hand Appeal: Soft hands with well-manicured short to medium-length nails.

Harem Pants: Softly draped trousers tied or gathered at the ankle.

Hem Length: The length of the distance from the floor to the hemline.

Hemline: Where the hem around a garment is equal distance from the floor.

I

IBBers: People who practice inner beauty being—their beauty radiates from the inside out.

Image: The way in which a person or thing is popularly perceived or regarded—public impression.

Image Power: Personal power that is derived from displaying a legitimate, poised and polished image.

Inner Beauty Being: A person whose beauty radiates from the inside out. Also, the acts and expressions of such a person.

J

Jersey: Stretchy fine-knitted fabric, used in tee-shirts and sportswear and figure-hugging garments; especially good for draping.

Jewel Neck: A simple round neckline at the base of the neck.

Jodhpur: Trousers worn for horse riding, very full from hip to knee and tight over the calf; finished with a piece of elastic under the foot.

Jumpsuit: An all-in-one garment with bodice and pants joined.

K

Keyhole: A round neckline with an inverted wedge or oval-shaped opening at the front.

Kick Pleat: A pleated plaid skirt with an unpleated panel in the front.

Kimono: A Japanese coat-like garment, obi-sash belted with long wide rectangular sleeves. Fabrics used are often luxurious and highly decorated.

Knife Pleat: A very narrow pleat pressed to form regular sharp pleats to skirts and dresses.

L

Lamé: A luxurious and shiny fabric made with either gold or silver metallic threads.

Lantern Sleeve: A bell sleeve with the wrist section joining at the bottom; the shape resembles a lantern.

Lapel: The front part of a garment that turns back and folds back to form a continuation of a collar.

Line: An effect, outline or style that is given by the construction and cut of a garment.

Lingerie: A woman's lightweight underclothing.

Lounge Wear: Clothing that is worn while lounging.

Low-Rise: Style for skirts and pants where the waistband fits low on the hip rather than on the waist.

Lycra: A man-made stretch fabric made from elasticized yarns, an essential component in underwear and other figure-hugging garments, especially sportswear.

M

Mandarin: A small standing collar that hugs the neck.

Maribou: A fur-like trim made from feather remnants, a smaller version of the boa, popular in dress-trimming for eveningwear.

Mary Jane: Flat or low-heeled ladies' shoe with a buttoned ankle-strap fastening.

Maxiskirt: A long full-length skirt.

MFBC: The media, fashion and beauty connection.

Miniskirt: A short skirt that falls at mid-thigh.

Monochromatic: Dressing in one color from head to toe.

Motif: A design used as a pattern or decoration.

N

Negligee: A decorative dressing gown.

O

Obi: A wide Japanese sash belt worn with a kimono.

Opaque: Non-transparent.

Over Blouse: A blouse that is untucked at the waistline.

Over-Sized: An enlarged garment, altering the natural silhouette of the wearer.

Over Skirt: A decorative skirt worn over another garment.

P

Paillette: A small piece of metal—a spangle used to ornament a dress or costume.

Pantsuit: A woman's suit consisting of pants and a jacket.

Parker: Padded hooded anorak-style coat. Often fur trims the hood. Popular in shades of green, navy and brown.

Patchwork: Technique of sewing pieces of fabric together to form a larger piece.

Patent: A high-gloss and waterproof finishing to leather and nylon.

Peep Toe: Popular shoe style where the front section is cut away to reveal the wearer's toes.

Pencil Skirt: Popular skirt shape cut from a straight block from hip to hem. Often knee-length and worn with suit jackets.

Peasant Sleeve: A full sleeve set into a dropped shoulder, which is usually gathered into a wristband.

Peplum: A small flounce or extension of a garment around the hips; usually from a bodice.

Perfect: Having all the qualities or elements that are necessary to its nature or kind. You!

Peter Pan Collar: A small flat shaped collar with two equal rounded lapels indented in the middle.

Placket: A garment opening which is fastened with a zipper, buttons, snaps or hooks and eyes.

Plunge: A neckline that is cut so low that it reveals the curve of the breast.

Polo Shirt: A short-sleeved pullover with a small flat collar.

Poncho: Traditionally a circular piece of fabric with a hole cut away for the head. Acts as a cape/jacket and is more often knitted with tassels.

Princess Line: A fitted dress where the skirt and bodice are fitted with vertical seams instead of darts.

Puffball: A double-layered skirt that stands out from the body and has a padded look to it.

Pussy Bow: A large bow that usually ties around the neck; can also be added as a detail to the waist and wrist.

Q

Quilted: A padding technique enclosing a layer of wadding between two pieces of fabric, held in place by sewing a diamond pattern over fabrics.

R

Ribbing: A knitting technique where small rows are finely knitted together to form a texture.

Ruche/Ruched: ("roosh") Fabric gathered and sewn into a seam shorter than the length of the fabric. Often used for trim but also used to create draping and texture within the body of the garment.

S

Sash: An ornamental band or scarf worn around the waist.

Sateen: A thicker version of satin, with a thicker weave; very luxurious for eveningwear and linings of jackets.

Satin: Fabric of a particular weave and gloss finish. The finish is achieved by heat treatment, resulting in a fabric with a high sheen face and matt reverse side. Often but not exclusively made from silk; modern alternatives include rayon.

Scalloped: Fabric or material cut into semicircles at the border or edge.

Scoop: A deep neckline cut in the shape of a U.

Seersucker: A lightweight cotton, rayon or silk fabric with a crinkled striped surface.

Selfing Process: The communication of the self, which allows you to *put on*—to present an authentic image or persona to the world.

Shawl: A triangular piece of fabric worn around the shoulders.

Sheath: A close-fitting dress with a straight skirt.

Sheer: A transparent fabric.

Shift: A simple unstructured dress slightly fitted at the bust with darts and clean lines down to the knee.

Shirtwaist: A dress with a bodice that has details similar to a shirt.

Silhouette: The outline of a figure or garment.

Single-Breasted: A center front closure with enough flap to accommodate one row of buttons.

Slit: A long and narrow opening.

Slogans: Wordage covering the front of a tee-shirt or dress.

Spaghetti Straps: Very fine, ribbon-like dress straps, popular on summer dresses.

Spandex: A popular sportswear fabric often used in swimwear, leotards and hosiery.

Split Image: Dressing in a poised and polished manner while speaking and acting in an unrefined manner. Or vice versa.

Stole: A long scarf that is wrapped around the shoulders.

Sunburst Pleats: Fine knife pleats that burst out from the waistband of a skirt, similar in shape to a sunray.

Surplice: A bodice with one side wrapping over the other side.

T

Tailor: A person who makes and/or alters clothes and fashions according to your body's specifications.

Train: An extended part of a garment which trails down the back, as on a wedding gown.

Trench Coat: A military-styled rainproof coat with many details—pockets, flaps and sometimes epaulettes, usually buttoned and tied with a belt of same fabric.

Tulle: A very fine mesh like net fabric, used in eveningwear and bridal gowns.

Tunic: A long top that extends below the waist and is usually worn over a lower garment.

Turtleneck: A high turnover collar that hugs the throat.

Tweed: A soft thick fabric, woven from contrasting woolen yarns, popular for coats and suits.

V

V-Neck: A neckline shaped in front like the letter V.

Velour: A soft material similar to velvet used for tracksuits and other sportswear items.

Velvet: Closely woven short pile fabric, soft and rich to touch.

Vest: A short close-fitting sleeveless garment.

W

Word Power: Having the ability to communicate effectively with vivid, expressive and colorful language.

Wrap Around: A garment or part of a garment that is wrapped around the body, such as a dress, skirt or cape.

Y

Yoke: A fitted portion of a garment, usually at the hips or shoulders, which is designed to support the rest of a garment hanging from it.

Printed in the United States
74410LV00004B/289-348